Community-Based Health Literacy Interventions

PROCEEDINGS OF A WORKSHOP

Joe Alper, *Rapporteur*

Roundtable on Health Literacy

Board on Population Health and Public Health Practice

Health and Medicine Division

The National Academies of
SCIENCES · ENGINEERING · MEDICINE

THE NATIONAL ACADEMIES PRESS
Washington, DC
www.nap.edu

THE NATIONAL ACADEMIES PRESS 500 Fifth Street, NW Washington, DC 20001

This activity was supported by contracts between the National Academy of Sciences and AbbVie Inc.; Aetna Foundation; Agency for Healthcare Research and Quality (HHSP23337024); American Dental Association; Bristol-Myers Squibb; East Bay Community Foundation (Kaiser Permanente); Eli Lilly and Company; Health Literacy Media; Health Literacy Partners; Health Resources and Services Administration (HHSH25034011T); Humana; Institute for Healthcare Advancement; Merck Sharpe & Dohme Corp.; National Institutes of Health (HHSN26300054); National Library of Medicine; New York University Langone Health System; Northwell Health; Office of Disease Prevention and Health Promotion (HHSP23337043); and UnitedHealth Group. Any opinions, findings, conclusions, or recommendations expressed in this publication do not necessarily reflect the views of any organization or agency that provided support for the project.

International Standard Book Number-13: 978-0-309-46667-7
International Standard Book Number-10: 0-309-46667-9
Digital Object Identifier: https://doi.org/10.17226/24917

Additional copies of this publication are available for sale from the National Academies Press, 500 Fifth Street, NW, Keck 360, Washington, DC 20001; (800) 624-6242 or (202) 334-3313; http://www.nap.edu.

Printed in the United States of America

Suggested citation: National Academies of Sciences, Engineering, and Medicine. 2018. *Community-based health literacy interventions: Proceedings of a workshop*. Washington, DC: The National Academies Press. doi: https://doi.org/10.17226/24917.

The National Academies of

SCIENCES · ENGINEERING · MEDICINE

The **National Academy of Sciences** was established in 1863 by an Act of Congress, signed by President Lincoln, as a private, nongovernmental institution to advise the nation on issues related to science and technology. Members are elected by their peers for outstanding contributions to research. Dr. Marcia McNutt is president.

The **National Academy of Engineering** was established in 1964 under the charter of the National Academy of Sciences to bring the practices of engineering to advising the nation. Members are elected by their peers for extraordinary contributions to engineering. Dr. C. D. Mote, Jr., is president.

The **National Academy of Medicine** (formerly the Institute of Medicine) was established in 1970 under the charter of the National Academy of Sciences to advise the nation on medical and health issues. Members are elected by their peers for distinguished contributions to medicine and health. Dr. Victor J. Dzau is president.

The three Academies work together as the **National Academies of Sciences, Engineering, and Medicine** to provide independent, objective analysis and advice to the nation and conduct other activities to solve complex problems and inform public policy decisions. The National Academies also encourage education and research, recognize outstanding contributions to knowledge, and increase public understanding in matters of science, engineering, and medicine.

Learn more about the National Academies of Sciences, Engineering, and Medicine at **www.nationalacademies.org**.

The National Academies of
SCIENCES • ENGINEERING • MEDICINE

Consensus Study Reports published by the National Academies of Sciences, Engineering, and Medicine document the evidence-based consensus on the study's statement of task by an authoring committee of experts. Reports typically include findings, conclusions, and recommendations based on information gathered by the committee and the committee's deliberations. Each report has been subjected to a rigorous and independent peer-review process and it represents the position of the National Academies on the statement of task.

Proceedings published by the National Academies of Sciences, Engineering, and Medicine chronicle the presentations and discussions at a workshop, symposium, or other event convened by the National Academies. The statements and opinions contained in proceedings are those of the participants and are not endorsed by other participants, the planning committee, or the National Academies.

For information about other products and activities of the National Academies, please visit www.nationalacademies.org/about/whatwedo.

PLANNING COMMITTEE ON COMMUNITY-BASED HEALTH LITERACY INTERVENTIONS[1]

STEVEN TEUTSCH (*Chair*), Adjunct Professor, Fielding School of Public Health, University of California, Los Angeles
LAURIE FRANCIS, Senior Director of Clinic Operations and Quality, Oregon Primary Care Association
ROMANA HASNAIN-WYNIA, Chief Research Officer, Denver Health
ANDREW PLEASANT, Senior Advisor on Health Literacy Interventions, Research, and Evaluation, Health Literacy Media
EARNESTINE WILLIS, Kellner Professor in Pediatrics, Medical College of Wisconsin

[1] The National Academies of Sciences, Engineering, and Medicine's planning committees are solely responsible for organizing the workshop, identifying topics, and choosing speakers. The responsibility for the published Proceedings of a Workshop rests with the workshop rapporteur and the institution.

ROUNDTABLE ON HEALTH LITERACY[1]

BERNARD ROSOF (*Chair*), Professor of Medicine, Donald and Barbara Zucker School of Medicine at Hofstra/Northwell, and CEO, QHC Advisory Group, LLC
WILMA ALVARADO-LITTLE, Principal and Founder, Alvarado-Little Consulting, LLC
SUZANNE BAKKEN, Alumni Professor of Nursing and Professor of Biomedical Informatics, Columbia University
CINDY BRACH, Senior Health Policy Researcher, Agency for Healthcare Research and Quality
GEMIRALD DAUS, Public Health Analyst, Office of Health Equity, Health Resources and Services Administration
TERRY C. DAVIS, Professor of Medicine and Pediatrics, Louisiana State University Health Sciences Center
CHRISTOPHER DEZII, Director, Healthcare Quality and Performance Measures, Bristol-Myers Squibb
JENNIFER DILLAHA, Medical Director for Immunizations, Medical Advisor, Health Literacy and Communication, Arkansas Department of Health
JAMES DUHIG, Head, Risk Communication and Behavioral Systems, Office of Patient Safety, AbbVie Inc.
WILLIAM ELWOOD, OppNet/Health Scientist Administrator, National Institutes of Health
ALICIA FERNANDEZ, Professor of Clinical Medicine, Department of Medicine, Division of General Internal Medicine, University of California, San Francisco
LAURIE FRANCIS, Senior Director of Clinic Operations and Quality, Oregon Primary Care Association
LORI HALL, Director, Health Literacy, U.S. Medical Strategy and Operations, Lilly USA, LLC
LINDA HARRIS, Director, Division of Health Communication and eHealth Team, U.S. Department of Health and Human Services
JOAN KELLY, Chief Patient Experience Officer, New York University Langone Health System
LAURIE MYERS, Global Health Literacy Director, Merck Sharp & Dohme Corp.
CATINA O'LEARY, President and Chief Executive Officer, Health Literacy Media

[1] The National Academies of Sciences, Engineering, and Medicine's forums and roundtables do not issue, review, or approve individual documents. The responsibility for the published Proceedings of a Workshop rests with the workshop rapporteur and the institution.

MARYLYNN OSTROWSKI, Executive Director, Aetna Foundation
MICHAEL K. PAASCHE-ORLOW, Professor of Medicine, Boston University School of Medicine
TERRI ANN PARNELL, Principal and Founder, Health Literacy Partners
KIM PARSON, Strategic Consultant, Proactive Care Strategies, Humana
KAVITA PATEL, Managing Director for Clinical Transformation and Delivery, The Brookings Institution
ANDREW PLEASANT, Senior Advisor on Health Literacy Interventions, Research, and Evaluation, Health Literacy Media
LINDSEY A. ROBINSON, Thirteenth District Trustee, American Dental Association
STACEY ROSEN, Associate Professor of Cardiology, Donald and Barbara Zucker School of Medicine at Hofstra/Northwell, and Vice President, Women's Health, The Katz Institute for Women's Health
RIMA RUDD, Senior Lecturer on Health Literacy, Education, and Policy, Harvard T.H. Chan School of Public Health
STEVEN RUSH, Director, Health Literacy Innovations, UnitedHealth Group
MICHAEL VILLAIRE, Chief Executive Officer, Institute for Healthcare Advancement
EARNESTINE WILLIS, Kellner Professor in Pediatrics, Medical College of Wisconsin
AMANDA WILSON, Head, National Network Coordinating Office, National Library of Medicine
MICHAEL S. WOLF, Professor, Medicine and Learning Sciences, Associate Division Chief, Research Division of General Internal Medicine, Feinberg School of Medicine, Northwestern University
WINSTON F. WONG, Medical Director, Disparities Improvement and Quality Initiatives, Kaiser Permanente

Consultant

RUTH PARKER, Professor of Medicine, Pediatrics, and Public Health, Emory University School of Medicine

Health and Medicine Division Staff

LYLA HERNANDEZ, Senior Program Officer
MELISSA FRENCH, Program Officer
ALEXIS WOJTOWICZ, Senior Program Assistant
ROSE MARIE MARTINEZ, Senior Board Director, Board on Population Health and Public Health Practice

Reviewers

This Proceedings of a Workshop was reviewed in draft form by individuals chosen for their diverse perspectives and technical expertise. The purpose of this independent review is to provide candid and critical comments that will assist the National Academies of Sciences, Engineering, and Medicine in making each published proceedings as sound as possible and to ensure that it meets the institutional standards for quality, objectivity, evidence, and responsiveness to the charge. The review comments and draft manuscript remain confidential to protect the integrity of the process.

We thank the following individuals for their review of this proceedings:

SHARON E. BARRETT, Association of Clinicians for the Underserved
CHIMENE CASTOR, Howard University
AMANDA WILSON, National Library of Medicine

Although the reviewers listed above provided many constructive comments and suggestions, they were not asked to endorse the content of the proceedings nor did they see the final draft before its release. The review of this proceedings was overseen by **DAVID R. CHALLONER,** University of Florida. He was responsible for making certain that an independent examination of this proceedings was carried out in accordance with standards of the National Academies and that all review comments were carefully considered. Responsibility for the final content rests entirely with the rapporteur and the National Academies.

Acknowledgments

The sponsors of the National Academies of Sciences, Engineering, and Medicine's Roundtable on Health Literacy made it possible to plan and conduct the workshop on community-based health literacy interventions, which this publication summarizes. Federal sponsors included the Agency for Healthcare Research and Quality; Health Resources and Services Administration; National Institutes of Health; National Library of Medicine; and Office of Disease Prevention and Health Promotion at the U.S. Department of Health and Human Services. Non-federal sponsorship was provided by AbbVie Inc.; Aetna Foundation; American Dental Association; Bristol-Myers Squibb; East Bay Community Foundation (Kaiser Permanente); Eli Lilly and Company; Health Literacy Media; Health Literacy Partners; Humana; Institute for Healthcare Advancement; Merck Sharp & Dohme Corp.; New York University Langone Health System; Northwell Health; and UnitedHealth Group.

The roundtable would like to thank each of the moderators, panelists, reactors, and speakers for their time and effort. Moderators, panelists, reactors, and speakers were, in alphabetical order, Cynthia Baur, Cindy Brach, Maureen Daniels, William Elwood, Michele Erikson, Oscar Espinosa, Leslie Gelders, Ariella Herman, S. Marisa New, Catina O'Leary, Andrew Pleasant, Anil Thota, Michael Villaire, Sherrie Flynt Wallington, Earnestine Willis, and Caroline Young.

Contents

Boxes, Figures, and Tables

BOXES

FIGURES

TABLES

Acronyms and Abbreviations

ACA	Patient Protection and Affordable Care Act
CBPR	community-based participatory research
CDC	Centers for Disease Control and Prevention
CHW	community health worker
FQHC	federally qualified health center
HCI	Health Care Institute
MHFA	mental health first aid
RCT	randomized controlled trial
RE-AIM	Research, Effectiveness, Adoption, Implementation, and Maintenance
REALM	Rapid Estimate of Adult Literacy in Medicine
S-TOFHLA	Short Test of Functional Health Literacy in Adults
UCLA	University of California, Los Angeles

1

Introduction

In its landmark report, *Health Literacy: A Prescription to End Confusion* (IOM, 2004), the Institute of Medicine[1] noted that there are 90 million adults in the United States with limited health literacy who cannot fully benefit from what the health and health care systems have to offer. This report also stated that "improving individual health literacy requires great effort from the public health and health care systems, the education system, and society overall" (IOM, 2004, p. xiv). Since the release of that report, health literacy has become a vibrant research field that has developed and disseminated a wide range of tools and practices that have helped organizations ranging in size from large health care systems to individual health care providers and pharmacists to engage in health literate discussions with and provide health literate materials for patients and family members. Improving the health literacy of organizations can be an important component of addressing the social determinants of health and achieving the triple aim of improving the patient experience, improving the health of populations, and reducing the cost of care. However, the focus on organizations does not address the larger issue of how to improve health literacy across the U.S. population. Realizing that goal requires a larger effort, one that addresses health literacy at the community and population levels. To get a better understanding of the state of community-based health literacy

[1] As of March 2016, the Health and Medicine Division of the National Academies of Sciences, Engineering, and Medicine continues the consensus studies and convening activities previously carried out by the Institute of Medicine (IOM). The IOM name is used to refer to publications issued prior to July 2015.

BOX 1-1
Statement of Task

An ad hoc committee will plan and conduct a 1-day public workshop that will feature invited presentations and discussion of community-based health literacy interventions. Potential areas of focus include the range of community-based health literacy interventions that currently exist, research related to community-based health literacy interventions, and best practices in community-based health literacy interventions.

The workshop will also include the presentation of a commissioned paper on community-based health literacy interventions. The committee will define the specific topics to be addressed, develop the agenda, and select and invite speakers and other participants. A proceedings of the workshop will be prepared by a designated rapporteur in accordance with institutional guidelines.

interventions, the Roundtable on Health Literacy hosted a workshop on community-based health literacy interventions. This workshop, organized by an ad hoc planning committee (see Box 1-1), was held on July 19, 2017. It featured examples of community-based health literacy programs, discussions on how to evaluate such programs, and the actions the field can take to embrace this larger view of health literacy. To help inform the discussions at the workshop, the roundtable also commissioned a review of community-based health literacy interventions and their outcomes that have been reported in the literature (see Appendix C).

ORGANIZATION OF THE PROCEEDINGS OF A WORKSHOP

An independent planning committee organized this workshop in accordance with the procedures of the National Academies of Sciences, Engineering, and Medicine. (See Appendix A for the workshop agenda.) The planning committee's members were Steven Teutsch (Chair), Laurie Francis, Romana Hasnain-Wynia, Andrew Pleasant, and Earnestine Willis. This publication summarizes the workshop's presentations and discussions, and it highlights the reactions to the proposed framework from a broad range of stakeholders, which will inform preparation of the roadmap for integrating health literacy, cultural competency, and language access services into a revised measurement framework. Chapter 2 discusses the methods used to conduct the commissioned literature review and the results of that review. Chapter 3 describes several community-based health literacy programs and Chapter 4 focuses on the issues and challenges in evaluating community-based health literacy programs. Chapter 5 recounts a moderated discussion on where the field needs to go in the future, and Chapter 6 summarizes the roundtable members' reflections on the day's discussions.

In accordance with the policies of the National Academies, the workshop did not attempt to establish any conclusions or recommendations about needs and future directions, focusing instead on issues identified by the speakers and workshop participants. In addition, the organizing committee's role was limited to planning the workshop. This Proceedings of a Workshop was prepared by workshop rapporteur Joe Alper as a factual summary of what occurred at the workshop.

2

Presentation and Discussion on the Commissioned Paper[1]

The workshop opened with Cynthia Baur, director of the Herschel S. Horowitz Center for Health Literacy at the University of Maryland School of Public Health, discussing the findings of the literature review she and her colleagues conducted, as well as the methodology they used to identify studies to include in the review (see Appendix C for the full paper). She began her presentation with what she called the "big idea" in the review paper: Many people are looking seriously at communities in need and trying to do something to help those communities get better information, build their skills, and become more health literate. "That being said, we know that good intentions are not enough," said Baur, "and we are here to discuss the science, the rigor of the design, and whether those were the right interventions." Despite the fact that many of the studies she and her colleagues identified might have had quality or scientific issues, she hoped the commissioned paper provided a sense of the richness of what she and her collaborators found in the literature.

After acknowledging her three co-authors—Lourdes Martinez from the Centers for Disease Control and Prevention (CDC), librarian Nedelina Tchangalova from the University of Maryland, and Don Rubin from the University of Georgia—as well as two other colleagues from CDC—Tom Chapel and Dogan Erglu—who were instrumental in choosing an evalu-

[1] This section is based on the presentation by Cynthia Baur, director of the Herschel S. Horowitz Center for Health Literacy at the University of Maryland School of Public Health, and the statements are not endorsed or verified by the National Academies of Sciences, Engineering, and Medicine.

ation framework, she listed the three questions that shaped the review as the review team began looking at the literature. The first question—What does it mean to take community seriously?—aimed to understand how community was identified in a study beyond merely the location. "We know that community has a much richer and broader meaning than just a location, but for many of the interventions, that was indeed the starting place," explained Baur.

The second question—What distinguishes a health literacy intervention from an educational intervention?—was important because the team had to sort through a rich literature of educational interventions to find studies that specifically tried to grapple with health literacy. The third question—What is or could be the "value added" element of doing a health literacy intervention with a community?—aimed to identify what health literacy brought to the many community interventions that focused on knowledge and building skills related to specific health concerns or health topics. CDC, she noted, has made huge investments in community-based work, and the health literacy issues were often not obvious to the funders, program planners, and evaluators. In Baur's opinion, there is valuable discussion to be had about what health literacy can bring to the work conducted under the rubric of community intervention. "How do we, as a field, help articulate that and increase the rigor and robustness of that work?" she asked.

With regard to the findings of the review, Baur chose to describe one of the two projects that had the greatest large-scale effects. The study she discussed, published in 2013, used a fotonovela developed at the Columbia School of Social Work (Hernandez and Organista, 2013) as the intervention vehicle. The study's intended outcomes were to increase literacy about depression, decrease the stigma associated with depression, and increase help seeking, knowledge, and beneficial behaviors. The investigators developed the fotonovela using social-cognitive theory, culture-centric narratives, and a definition of health literacy espoused by David Baker at Northwestern University (Baker, 2006). One group of participants received the fotonovela as the health literacy tool while a control group engaged in a group discussion about family communication issues led by promotoras[2] at a local community clinic for Latinas. The investigators designed the study as a pre- and posttest randomized experiment to test depression knowledge. The study included a health literacy score, measured using the Short Test of Functional Health Literacy in Adults (S-TOFHLA), but did not report a pre- and posttest assessment of health literacy. The results of the experiment showed a

[2] A promotora is a community health worker who is trained to provide basic health education within her community. More information is available at https://mhpsalud.org/programs/who-are-promotoresas-chws (accessed January 11, 2018).

large effect on stigma and intent to seek treatment and a moderate effect on self-efficacy to seek treatment for depression.

Discussing the broader findings and conclusions from the entire body of work that she and her colleagues examined, Baur said they found a wide range of interventions reporting a mix of qualitative and quantitative evidence, with a heavy emphasis on qualitative results. The papers mentioned the terms "health literacy" and "community" frequently, though often without defining those terms. One finding that Baur said emerged organically from the review was a pattern in the way that interventions used health literacy. Researchers, for example, selected people for the intervention based on either an assumed or documented low level of health literacy. They tried to measure something about health literacy in their evaluations using tools such as the Rapid Estimate of Adult Literacy in Medicine (REALM), S-TOFHLA, the Newest Vital Sign (Powers et al., 2010), a single question—do you feel comfortable with forms? (Chew et al., 2008)—or instruments they developed themselves. The studies used health literacy to help shape the actual intervention and it was often listed as an outcome. "This is something we labeled as a finding because we saw it consistently as a pattern across the interventions," said Baur. She also noted that the overall quality of the evidence in the publications could have been better.

One of the challenges to conducting this review was defining community, and Baur noted that the definition was a "moving target." She and her colleagues decided to use a published definition (McLeroy et al., 2003) that gave community four meanings: setting, the target population, a resource or asset, and an agent where the community is engaged in whatever issue it is being asked to consider. Setting and target population were the most frequent uses of the term "community." For example, publications would mention community hospitals, community clinics, or community agencies without defining the community element, or they would state that recruitment occurred in a community or that there were community participants without defining the boundaries of the community being studied. Community could also be defined by language, shared experience, or a combination of factors. "Communities were very challenging, and given our charge to find and talk about community-based health literacy interventions, we had to grapple with this concept throughout the review process," said Baur.

When describing the methods used to conduct the review, Baur noted the important role the team's professional research librarian played in maintaining the rigor of what she called a "scoping review." The purpose of a scoping review is to identify a broad area that provides an overall picture of a field of study while allowing for different study designs and mapping key concepts, sources, and types of evidence. A systematic review, by contrast, uses much tighter definitions about the types of studies to consider and focuses more on analyzing the quality of the evidence in the identified studies. The scoping review, Baur added, could serve as a prelude for conducting a systematic review at some point.

The professional librarian constructed and executed the search strategy, which included 14 commercial library databases and the Web-based "gray" literature. "Health literacy" and "community" were key search terms, with health literacy defined as both how people find, process, understand, and communicate about health information and services to protect and promote their health, and how organizations and systems support or hinder people in these activities. A community-based health literacy intervention was defined as any purposeful, organized activity to help a group of people find, understand, use, or communicate about health information, services, or issues for themselves or their communities.

For an evaluation framework, Baur and her colleagues used a modified version of the CDC Best Practices Framework, which looks at applied public health interventions and evaluates them based on five dimensions: effectiveness, reach, feasibility, sustainability, and transferability (Spencer et al., 2013). She noted that they found some information about effectiveness and reach in the papers they identified, but very little about feasibility, sustainability, and transferability, which are factors that would be important for scaling and spreading an intervention. They did multiple rounds of review, starting with titles and abstracts before moving to a full-text review, and then developed a list of reporting categories to organize the results (see Box 2-1).

BOX 2-1
Categories Used to Organize the Results of the Literature Review

- Health literacy skill and capacity building
- Information seeking
- Culturally sensitive
- Adult learners
- Early childhood
- Schools
- Other
- Chronic disease
- Mental health
- Medicines
- Cancer
- Environmental health
- Policy/system

SOURCE: As presented by Cynthia Baur at the Community-Based Health Literacy Interventions workshop on July 19, 2017.

Table 2-1 lists the inclusion and exclusion criteria Baur and her colleagues used to initially identify 2,402 papers. They reduced the list to 140 papers for full-text review and 74 papers for inclusion in their analysis. Review articles, she noted, were a source of additional references to check, but the review articles themselves were excluded from the analysis. She explained that the full-text review revealed frequent superficial uses of health literacy in abstracts, but little or no uses of health literacy in the actual intervention. As she noted earlier, only two papers—the one she described on depression and a second one about a cancer screening program—reported large-scale effects.

In discussing the results, Baur said there were quite a few studies on health literacy skill and capacity building, mostly from outside of the United States, and a few on information seeking, mostly led by librarians who were trying to build people's information-seeking skills. Several studies had the specific goal of creating culturally sensitive or culturally targeted interventions, while studies in other categories included cultural sensitivity as an aspect. A handful of studies were about adult learners enrolled in formal programs offered through adult literacy organizations or at a community college, and other studies focused on Head Start programs. Some

TABLE 2-1 Inclusion and Exclusion Criteria for the Literature Review

Inclusion	Exclusion
1. Published in English	1. Conceptual models
2. Published between June 2010–2017	2. Associations between health literacy and another concept or variable
3. Peer-reviewed articles (exceptions are theses, dissertations, Web pages, posters, and professional/trade publications when enough information was included)	3. Intervention development or protocols
4. Used a community sample	4. Formative research
5. "Health literacy" and "community" common terms	5. Interventions focused on health care professionals or individuals (not groups)
	6. Questionnaire or other instrument development
	7. "Health literacy" and "community" absent in abstract
	8. Health knowledge or skills without a health literacy connection
	9. Community locations or settings, such as health center, used only for recruitment
	10. Review articles, but reference lists were searched for articles meeting inclusion criteria

SOURCE: Adapted from a presentation by Cynthia Baur at the Community-Based Health Literacy Interventions workshop on July 19, 2017.

studies were based in schools, although Baur said the number was fewer than expected, perhaps because schools are complicated institutions and not always easy to use as intervention sites.

Baur and her colleagues decided to include mental health as a category, even though previous reviews did not, because of the sheer number of interventions focused on mental health. "We decided that if there are researchers or practitioners in other fields invoking the term 'health literacy' or talking about what they do as health literacy, even if it does not mean the same thing to the people in this room today, it is still worth considering what they mean, what we mean, and how to engage with them," said Baur. The only paper on a policy or a system change included in the review came from Sweden, she said, and it was supposed to have implications for health literacy, but was not on a policy specific to health literacy. Reported outcomes in the 74 papers are listed in Box 2-2.

Four themes emerged from the review, said Baur. There was a strong community engagement component in all of the papers, which included formative research to identify community needs or to address health literacy issues in a community. The studies all had a health literacy intervention component, and a few papers made a link between health knowledge and health literacy. The commissioned paper also discussed the limitations of

BOX 2-2
Reported Outcomes in the 74 Reviewed Papers

- Satisfaction
- Knowledge
- Understanding
- Awareness
- Self-efficacy
- Intentions
- Attitudes/beliefs
- Self-management tasks
- Goals
- Health behaviors
- Decision making
- Information seeking
- Health services use
- Physical changes
- Health literacy (general)

SOURCE: As presented by Cynthia Baur at the Community-Based Health Literacy Interventions workshop on July 19, 2017.

the evaluation framework used in the studies, which she said might speak to the standards of different journals and what they expect investigators to report as far as the level of detail. To that point, she said it would be worth having a discussion about what level of detail should be reported in papers on health literacy interventions. "I think there is more information that people should be providing to all of us about what they are doing, not just for the sake of transparency, but also to understand how these effects they are reporting are happening," said Baur. "Much of that was really behind the curtain."

Referring back to the three questions that framed the review process, Baur said she and her colleagues have not developed a hard and fast definition of community that they would be willing to defend. Community, however, has to move beyond just the setting and target audience if the goal is to take community engagement seriously and move beyond the 100- to 300-person studies that were typical in the papers they reviewed. She also noted that more discussion is needed about the distinction between health literacy and health education, and not just at a definitional level. "It is more productive to think about [that distinction] in the light of the question about what do we bring to the table," said Baur. "How do we take what we have learned over the past 20 to 30 years about health literacy interventions and make that meaningful to people thinking they are doing health literacy interventions?" Her final comment was that many of the projects she and her colleagues reviewed would have had a bigger impact if they had looked at health literacy.

DISCUSSION

Rima Rudd from the Harvard T.H. Chan School of Public Health opened the discussion by asking Baur to explain why her team's review identified 74 papers describing community-based health literacy interventions while another group, headed by Don Nutbeam at the University of Sydney, found only seven articles for a review his team conducted 1 year earlier. Baur replied that she and her colleagues posed that question to the workshop planning committee when they first started their review process and asked for direction on how narrowly the planning committee wanted her team to define the field.

The Nutbeam group's framework, explained Baur, focused on functional, interactive, and critical health literacy and used health literacy as the outcome. Her team, taking direction from the planning committee, expanded its search criteria to include studies where health literacy was included at any point of an intervention. She noted that the seven papers Nutbeam identified used the terms "community" and "population" interchangeably. Her team, by contrast, used the term "community" exclusively and defined community as having some element of groupness as a means of distinguishing what they called individual and non-individual interventions. As an example of the former, she said that some studies reported recruiting from a population, delivering the intervention to individuals, and then aggregating and reporting the data in some manner. "For us, that was an exclusion criterion if an intervention functioned that way," said Baur. "There had to be some kind of group dynamic and some explanation of why the community was chosen." One element missing from the majority of the papers was an explanation of how interactions among the community members affected outcomes.

Michael Paasche-Orlow from Boston University complimented Baur for acknowledging the complexity of the term "community" and wondered if her team's definition of the word could have been even broader to include studies that are doing community-based research, but never use the term "community." Baur agreed that might be the case, but in the end, she and her colleagues had to set some operating rules. "Any method is going to choose some things and not choose others," said Baur. "We tried to be as transparent as possible about our methods." She added that her group took the same approach with the term "health literacy." Frequently, she said, papers would specifically mention health literacy in the title or abstract, but a closer reading of the paper failed to find the health literacy piece of the study.

Paasche-Orlow then asked Baur to comment on the observation that the way the 74 studies defined a community always focused their work on vulnerable or poor populations. "If these things work, why do we not use them on rich people?" he asked. Baur replied that the groups conducting those studies were looking at communities of greatest need. "If we are thinking about resource allocation, you could argue that resources are being allocated appropriately because they are going to the communities with the greatest need," said Baur. She explained that none of the 74 studies defined communities by socioeconomic status and none looked at whether the intervention was more or less successful in high versus medium versus low socioeconomic communities. Bernard Rosof from the Quality HealthCare Advisory Group and Northwell Health remarked that perhaps all communities could benefit from health literacy interventions, to which Baur responded, "They may need them, but who needs them more?" Most of the papers, she said, opened with statements concerning the high needs of the communities on which their work focused.

William Elwood from the National Institutes of Health commented that epidemiology is not the sole driver of health literacy. What people know is also a driver, and often what people know is inaccurate. To that point, he asked Baur why the search criteria did not include knowledge as an outcome. Baur replied that her group argued that knowledge should be considered an important outcome and it was considered an inclusion criterion.

Jennifer Dillaha from the Arkansas Department of Health said she agreed with Baur's decision to make a distinction between health education and health literacy because in her opinion, health literacy enables people to gain knowledge more easily from health education interventions. She then asked Baur if she considered whether interventions designed for specific chronic diseases are more about health education than health literacy. Baur said she and her colleagues struggled with that question when trying to decide whether to include studies focusing on mental health and nutrition. "We thought it was better to bring that body of work to you and ask what you think rather than exclude them," she said. "How do we feel about people parsing this and talking about diabetes literacy and nutrition literacy and cancer literacy and all these variants, [including] mental health literacy? Do we think that is a good thing? Do we need to be partnering with them? Do they mean the same thing? If they mean something different, how do we engage them in what we mean?"

John Gardenier, recently retired from the National Center for Health Statistics, commented that this discussion was missing attention to affect or motivation. "People may have high or low health literacy, but if they have no motivation to apply health literacy to their own or to their community situation, it does not seem to be likely that there will be a strong positive outcome," said Gardenier. He also noted that people are defined by the parameters of a community, not necessarily by identifying with that community, and that a degree of affective identification with a community would have a great deal to do with the efficacy of a community intervention. Considering his second point reminded Baur of one study that provoked a great deal of discussion among her team. This dementia intervention involved three Aboriginal communities in Australia and the paper described how the intervention led the community to engage in discussion on a subject it had previously found difficult and to better understand what was causing some community members to act strangely. Clearly, said Baur, this intervention had a positive effect in the community, but she was unclear on how it was relevant to the type of effects the planning committee had asked her team to identify in their review.

Donney John from NOVA Scripts Central remarked that while sustainability was one of the five criteria for the review framework, Baur's team did not find much information about sustainability in the reviewed papers. He asked Baur if she and her colleagues came across any programs that successfully scaled their interventions or were unable to sustain them. Baur replied that one or two papers may have had a sustainability component, but most of the investigators were conducting traditional pilot studies that looked at outcomes.

John then asked whether incorporating studies focused on providers, who were excluded from this review, might have found more work on sustainability given that providers might get reimbursed for this type of activity, which could lead to sustainability. Baur responded that doing so would have required deciding whether to count every counseling intervention as a community intervention. For example, there was a diabetes intervention (Handley et al., 2016) that trained promotoras and community health workers to do individual follow-ups with people. Her team questioned whether to count a one-on-one counseling intervention as a community intervention and decided that the community aspect of the study involved recruitment, not the intervention itself. Similarly, they found three studies that focused on training students, such as dental and pharmacy students, but decided there was no community component to these interventions.

Turkan Gardenier from Pragmatica suggested adding the term "comprehensibility" to any measure of value added. Baur replied that this was why they included content in the four-part structure of the review. She added that studies were addressing comprehension issues with the way in which the content used in their interventions was designed. Baur noted that the commissioned paper listed several excluded publications in a section of the review called papers of interest because these publications talked about reporting the results of their interventions back to the community.

Elwood noted that a new rule will go into effect on January 1, 2018, that will require any human subjects study receiving National Institutes of Health funding to list all social and behavioral interventions and, eventually, all study protocols on their ClinicalTrials.gov posting. These requirements, he said, create a great route for disseminating information. "I think we are about to see a tremendous expansion of the availability of information and a much broader and also deepened discussion about research, its results, and diffusing it across all levels of the American people, not just the research community," said Elwood.

Ruth Parker from the Emory University School of Medicine said she knows of interventions that she would call "community-based" and related to health literacy that did not make the list of 74 publications Baur and her colleagues reviewed. "That makes me worried," said Parker, because the terms "health literacy" and "community" were not in the abstracts or titles of those papers. Parker also expressed concern that interventions that targeted specific conditions such as diabetes or mental illness may have been left out of the commissioned paper because the titles and abstracts did not contain those two specific phrases. Baur replied that the authors had to have some way of distinguishing a health literacy intervention from other types of interventions. Parker then asked Baur if she knew the impact factors of the journals that published the reviewed papers, and Baur replied that she and her colleagues did not track impact factor.

3

Examples of Community-Based Health Literacy Programs

The workshop's second session presented examples of community-based health literacy programs delivered in various settings and a panel discussion on implementing community-based health literacy interventions (see Box 3-1). Marisa New, board member of the Oklahoma Health Equity Network and chair of the Southwest Regional Health Equity Council, and Leslie Gelders, health literacy coordinator at the Oklahoma Department of Libraries, discussed community-based health literacy interventions in Oklahoma and included an example of a program focused on public libraries. Catina O'Leary, president and chief executive officer of Health Literacy Media, described health literacy activities in four communities in Missouri. Ariella Herman, research director at the Johnson & Johnson Health Care Institute and senior lecturer on decisions, operations, and technology management at the University of California, Los Angeles (UCLA), Anderson School of Management, reviewed health literacy interventions delivered through Head Start programs. Following the four presentations, Earnestine Willis, Kellner professor in pediatrics at the Medical College of Wisconsin, moderated a discussion with the panelists.

BOX 3-1
Suggestions from Speakers for Implementing Community-Based Health Literacy Interventions

- Partner with trusted organizations that are already operating within the community (Gelders, New, O'Leary).
- Choose locations for interventions that are known to the community and feel safe and comfortable (Gelders, Herman, New, O'Leary).
- Ask people in the community what they would like to see change with regard to their health and how they think that could be accomplished (Gelders, O'Leary).
- Provide people with information on the health status of their communities in ways that are easy to understand (Gelders, New).
- Adapt the intervention to reflect the context of each community (Gelders, Herman, O'Leary).

SOURCES: Adapted from presentations by Leslie Gelders, Ariella Herman, Marisa New, and Catina O'Leary at the Community-Based Health Literacy Interventions workshop on July 19, 2017.

HEALTH LITERACY IN PUBLIC LIBRARIES[1]

The Oklahoma Health Equity Campaign, which launched in 2008 and enhanced its focus on health literacy in 2011, is a grassroots coalition that aims to address the fact that Oklahoma has consistently been at the bottom of national health rankings, said Marisa New. In 2016, the United Health Foundation ranked Oklahoma as the 46th healthiest state, and the 2014 State of the State Health Report Card showed failing grades in the state's mortality rate, prevalence of diabetes, consumption of fresh fruits and vegetables, and physical activity. The state was also the sixth most obese state in the nation.

From its inception, the coalition has approached health equity from the perspective that there are many social determinants of health, said New, and it has conducted statewide surveys of communities to identify how community resources make an impact on health. The coalition has developed various position statements that highlight how life-enhancing

[1] This section is based on the presentation by Marisa New, board member of the Oklahoma Health Equity Network and chair of the Southwest Regional Health Equity Council, and Leslie Gelders, health literacy coordinator at the Oklahoma Department of Libraries, and the statements are not endorsed or verified by the National Academies of Sciences, Engineering, and Medicine.

community resources or social determinants, such as food security and public transportation, affect health.

In 2011, steering committee members recognized the value of having a library representative, and Leslie Gelders is now on the organization's board. In 2012, said New, Oklahoma had its first health literacy summit that it modeled after similar summits held in Florida and Wisconsin. The second summit, held in 2014, was called Health Literacy: A Powerful Tool for Prevention and Partnership, and it featured a dialogue session that helped the organization from a capacity-building perspective.

At a statewide coalition policy day in 2015, a session that focused on health literacy produced two policy recommendations. The first recommendation, New recounted, advocated for state leaders to understand the link between health and literacy and to reinstate funding for adult literacy programs. The other recommendation requested that the state legislature conduct an interim study examining the effects of low health literacy. In 2016, the coalition's health literacy action team, collaborating with more than two dozen public and private partners, provided evidence-based health literacy interventions such as Teach-Back and Ask Me 3. Nearly 100 individuals engaged in the training and then worked with decision makers from the public and private sectors to craft the Oklahoma Health Literacy Action Plan. The action plan called for the partner organizations to work to strengthen and sustainably support a home and infrastructure for the advancement of health literacy in Oklahoma. It also proposed coordinated statewide efforts to increase and evaluate efforts to address health literacy challenges or improve health literacy of Oklahoma residents. The coalition took advantage of Health Literacy Month in 2016 to share health literacy messages through social media and the Thunderclap social media amplifier, reaching more than 175,000 people.[2]

Unfortunately, said New, the coalition's engagement has been limited over the past year because of budget pressures that have limited public resources. The coalition's steering committee decided to forge ahead as a nonprofit organization and has since engaged with the Southwest Regional Health Equity Network, which serves Arkansas, Louisiana, New Mexico, Oklahoma, and Texas. In 2015, this network developed a blueprint for enhancing individual and community health, with the objective of launching a health literacy campaign that would align with the Robert Wood Johnson Foundation's Culture of Health framework and the National Action Plan to Improve Health Literacy, explained New. The Oklahoma team's strategy has been to focus on two evidence-based interventions: the Teach-Back method and Ask Me 3 approach.

---

[2] This exercise was repeated in October 2017; see https://twitter.com/search?q=%23healthliterateok&src=typd (accessed February 9, 2018).

Gelders then spoke about a specific health literacy program that the Oklahoma Department of Libraries started in 2012 after the first Oklahoma health literacy summit. With assistance and urging from Wisconsin Health Literacy, Gelders wrote a grant and received funds to launch this initiative at five pilot sites across the state. Addressing the question of why she focused on community-based health literacy activities in libraries, Gelders cited a 2015 Pew Research study showing that 73 percent of people who visited a public library in America went there looking for answers about their health. Another study by the Institute of Museum and Library Services showed that over a 12-month period, an estimated 28 million people used the public library to seek assistance from a librarian or to use resources and computers in the library to find out about health and wellness issues, including learning about their medical conditions and finding health care providers. "The question was, 'Why libraries?' and the answer is because people are already using their public library to find information about their health," said Gelders.

Libraries, she noted, are trusted community institutions that offer a non-threatening environment for all members of the community and serve as places of lifelong learning. One reason why libraries may be able to play an important role in health literacy efforts is that the computer and Internet services available at public libraries can provide access to reliable health information for people who do not have access to computers or the Internet elsewhere. In fact, said Gelders, 70 percent of rural public libraries are the only providers of free Internet in their communities. A second reason is that librarians are information experts and they offer their services for free. She noted that some public librarians are taking courses to become health information specialists, and some libraries have health-related tools such as blood pressure monitors, accurate scales, and pedometers for patrons to use.

Gelders remarked that since libraries already offer free programming on a number of topics for adults, teens, and children, it would be relatively easy to include health literacy, health, and wellness topics in that programming. Libraries, through their many connections in communities, can help promote health literacy efforts through their networks. Libraries may offer free space for health literacy programs, and they may have access to state or federal funds they can use for health literacy programming, said Gelders. One caveat, she said, is that many librarians do not know what health literacy means, so they may be intimidated by the thought of initiating a health literacy project or becoming a partner in such a project. One of her roles in Oklahoma has been to provide ideas, technical assistance, and support to libraries to address that problem.

With regard to the grant she procured, Gelders explained that each of the five pilot sites was asked to plan a project based on actual community needs as noted, in part, by their communities' scores on the State of the State Health Report. Many of the grantees focused their efforts on healthy eating and exercise, accessing and using credible health information, and providing community education through programming. One program in rural Healdton, Oklahoma, for example, was a hands-on project on healthy eating for children. Over the course of a summer-long pickle-making class at the library, the children learned why it was important to eat fruits and vegetables and why they should control their salt and sugar intake. A family and consumer sciences educator led the project, which had the children work in one of the gardens built between the public library and the county health department.

Another project, based in Elk City, Oklahoma, created a virtual Route 66 walk-a-thon, where individuals and teams were challenged to walk the distance between Chicago and Santa Monica, California, and record their virtual journey on a map in the library. Gelders said 60 individuals walked a total of 16,261 miles, and the local newspaper ran articles about the walk-a-thon that included information about the benefits of increased exercise. In a Claremore, Oklahoma, English-as-a-second-language class, learners used a health-related curriculum and real-world health materials as part of their language instruction, while the Moore Public Library offered free weekly Tai Chi classes. In every case, library sites were required to partner with other organizations in their community, as well as with local health departments. All told, more than 43 organizations, including the local councils on aging, dentists and doctors, food pantries, grocery stories, senior centers, and the National Network of Libraries of Medicine, partnered with libraries to promote health and wellness in communities across Oklahoma. The partners, said Gelders, provided instruction, in-kind services, resources, funding, awareness, and a wealth of ideas to help expand the projects locally.

Gelders mentioned that many public libraries get funds from the state library, which is where she works. She offered her assistance to anyone who wants to get state libraries involved in making health literacy a priority activity. She noted that she hoped to award 25–30 health literacy grants, up from the initial 5, to public libraries in Oklahoma. Gelders also noted that there is an educational website for librarians called WebJunction, which contains a section titled Health Happens at Libraries that includes information, webinars, and examples of how libraries can become involved in promoting health and health literacy.[3]

She ended her presentation with two quotes. The first came from a public librarian, who said, "Good health for the community has been a mission for me. I did not realize how poor our health was until I began looking at

[3] See https://www.webjunction.org for more information (accessed March 21, 2018).

the statistics. It is very important for libraries to address the needs of their communities and it is a great need in Oklahoma." The second quote came from an English-as-a-second-language student who said, "I lost 34 pounds as a result of my literacy program. Even though I am studying for citizenship and working on English, I like the weekly weighing on the scales in the literacy office. My tutor helps me record my weight and she helps me read information on walking and eating better. I am smiling because I can see the results."

COVER MISSOURI'S COMMUNITY HEALTH LITERACY PROGRAM[4]

When communities ask the Cover Missouri Coalition to talk to their residents in a responsive way about health interventions that are meaningful, they rarely ask for health literacy by name, even though much of what they want has all of the components of health literacy, said Catina O'Leary. She noted that she has seen all over the world that what people want is to learn how and where to get information on health and wellness, and without using the words, develop health literacy skills.

For the past 4 years, the Cover Missouri Coalition has been working with O'Leary and her colleagues on health insurance literacy. This effort has three goals: promoting quality health coverage for every Missourian; improving the health insurance literacy of Missourians; and lowering the rate of uninsured Missourians to 5 percent by the end of 2018. With regard to the last goal, O'Leary said there was no chance of meeting it given that Missouri's elected leadership chose not to expand Medicaid coverage under the Patient Protection and Affordable Care Act (ACA). Nonetheless, she said, the Cover Missouri Coalition has grown to include some 900 partners, and bimonthly coalition meetings routinely have 200 to 300 navigators, assisters, and other representatives of the partner organizations who ask hard questions stemming from their experience working on the ground in their communities. Health Literacy Media's role, she explained, has been to educate the partners about the tools of health literacy and to help them think about how they do their work.

For the first 3 years of this effort, O'Leary's team conducted what she called standard health literacy activities: creating health literate written materials for assisters and navigators, training frontline workers on verbal and written communications, and helping them make the materials they were using more accessible. Then, in year 3, O'Leary and others in the coalition realized that while it was important to continue the work on

[4] This section is based on the presentation by Catina O'Leary, president and chief executive officer of Health Literacy Media, and the statements are not endorsed or verified by the National Academies of Sciences, Engineering, and Medicine.

awareness and other aspects of the technical assistance that her organization provided to the partners, there were people who either could not afford insurance because they were in the coverage gap or simply refused to buy it for any number of personal reasons. What the coalition decided to do was take a step back from health insurance to focus on general health and wellness in the community. To enable that effort the Missouri Foundation for Health funded a pilot program to support four communities' knowledge about health and health care in whatever manner those communities wanted that help.

The pilot program, said O'Leary, aims to engage the community around health and health insurance through strategies that lower barriers to health, and in doing so, help people make informed choices for their family's health. One outcome of this effort might be to get more people to enroll as they come to understand the value of health insurance to their family's health, but at the least the hope was to help families be healthier. "Our framework was to meet these communities where they are and infuse health literacy," said O'Leary.

The planning process for working in a community went through four phases (see Figure 3-1). The early planning phase involved selecting the four communities based on a set of criteria and identifying tracking and evaluation measures. In the second phase, two staff members assigned to each of the four communities identified and engaged key stakeholders and gatekeepers and organized a planning meeting with those individuals. In the third phase, staff interviewed the key stakeholders and various community partners to identify community priorities. Phase four involved strategic activity planning that included developing program activities to address community-identified health priorities and to coordinate and implement those activities. The purpose of this complex process, O'Leary explained, was to bring these communities to a place where they wanted health literacy and health education and to provide them with a single contact point who could connect them to whatever resources they needed. For example, if a community wanted media training, one of the staff members assigned to that community would make the necessary arrangements. She noted that the Missouri Foundation for Health provided a mere $5,000 for each community, but that small amount of money forced communities to think hard about what they wanted to accomplish with those funds.

As to how the coalition chose the four pilot communities (see Figure 3-2), it started with the decision to select one community from each of the four Missouri Foundation for Health's service regions outside of the St. Louis region. They excluded the St. Louis region because of the wealth of resources already in place thanks to the three major universities and other organizations in that region that had their own ongoing activities. In each of the four service areas that were too far from St. Louis to

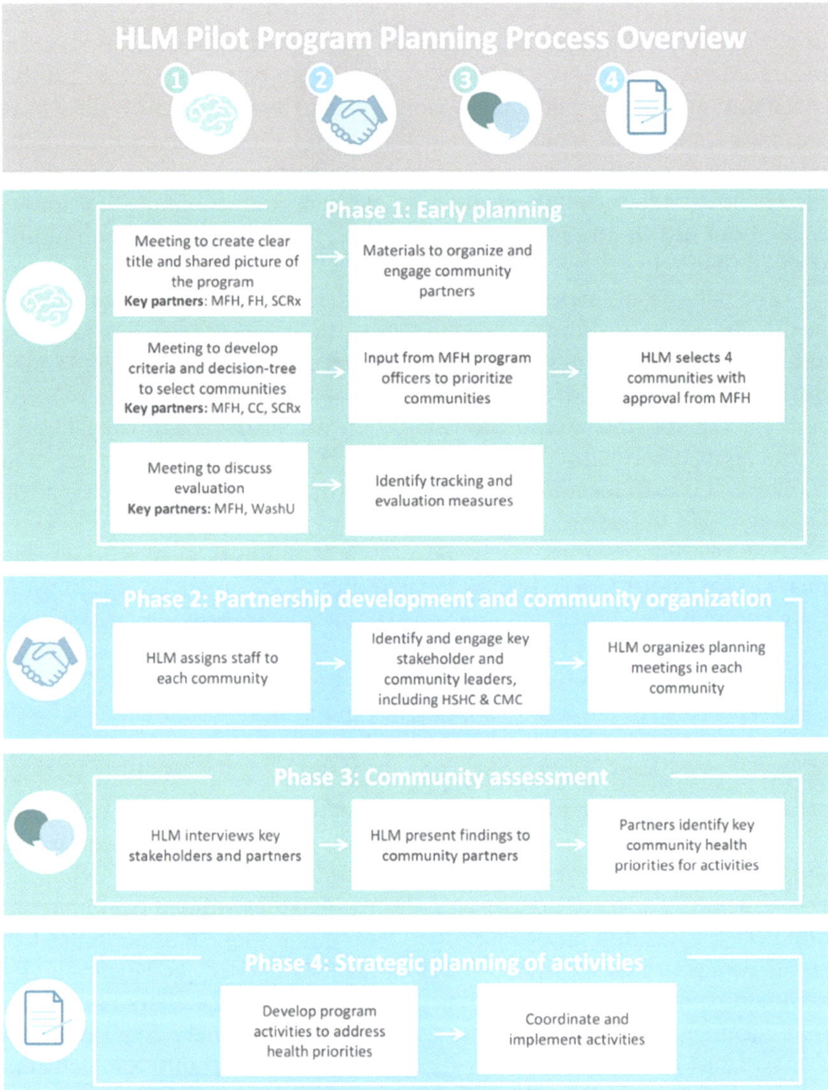

FIGURE 3-1 Health Literacy Media's (HLM's) pilot program planning process.
NOTE: CC = Community Catalyst; CMC = Cover Missouri Coalition; FH = FleishmanHillard; HSHC = Healthy Schools Healthy Communities; MFH = Missouri Foundation for Health; SCRx = StratCommRx; WashU = Washington University in St. Louis.
SOURCE: As presented by Catina O'Leary at the Community-Based Health Literacy Interventions workshop on July 19, 2017.

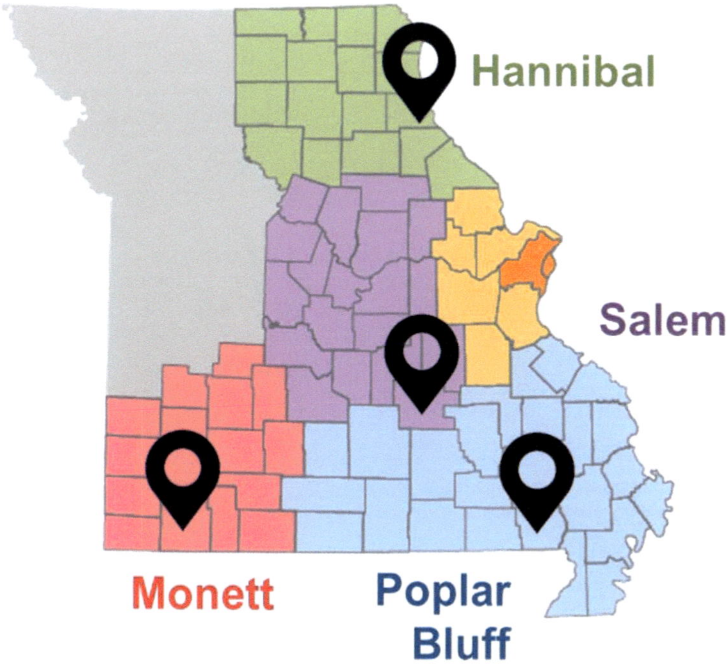

FIGURE 3-2 The four communities chosen for the pilot projects.
SOURCE: As presented by Catina O'Leary at the Community-Based Health Literacy Interventions workshop on July 19, 2017.

access those resources easily, the coalition identified communities in which 16 percent or more of the residents were uninsured and 18 percent or more had incomes below the Federal Poverty Level. Two other selection criteria were that the community included Missouri Foundation for Health priority populations and that there were some preexisting relationships with the community. "We did not want to go into communities that had nobody knowing anybody at all because we did not have enough time to start completely cold. We had to at least know one person at one organization who would say yes, please join us," explained O'Leary.

The final step in the selection process was to ask the communities to take part in the project and have the communities say yes. "We were fortunate that everybody selected us back, but we had to have a lot of meetings to ask a lot of people the question to make sure they selected us back before we started the work," said O'Leary. The four communities that said yes were Hannibal, Monett, Poplar Bluff, and Salem (see Table 3-1). They are mostly small communities with different levels of minority populations. Monett was of particular interest because it had a large population that did

TABLE 3-1 Demographics of the Four Pilot Communities

	Hannibal	Monett	Poplar Bluff	Salem
Population	17,717	8,957	17,195	4,976
Race	88.8% white 7.1% black 2.4% Hispanic	74.6% white 0.02% black 23.5% Hispanic	85.5% white 10.7% black 2.2% Hispanic	96% white 0.5% black 1.7% Hispanic
Education	82.4% high school diploma or higher	28% have at least some high school	78.9% high school diploma or higher	28% have at least some high school
Uninsured rate (for county)	16%	22%	17%	20%
Poverty rate	22.3%	28%	27.7%	33.3%

SOURCE: Adapted from a presentation by Catina O'Leary at the Community-Based Health Literacy Interventions workshop on July 19, 2017.

not speak English as its first language, and O'Leary was interested in how their interventions would work differently in such a population.

She noted that all of the communities have been great partners, but the Monett community was perhaps the most excited to be asked. One observation she made was that the Monett community was having difficulty applying for funding from foundations because of structural issues, such as the need for help even applying for a grant. "We have been able to bring some of those issues to light and start conversations about changing processes so communities like this that have a different level of vulnerability are not overlooked," said O'Leary.

As an aside, O'Leary said that a question people ask her is how she and her colleagues know that the selected communities have issues with health literacy. One answer is that 9 out of 10 Americans have a health literacy problem, but with regard to the selected communities, the answer is that they are comparatively undereducated, have high levels of poverty, and have high rates of uninsured community members.

With regard to what Health Literacy Media and the Cover Missouri Coalition provided to the chosen communities, O'Leary listed the following activities:

- Met with and interviewed partners in each community to hear their opinions on the health of their community;

- Conducted media and awareness efforts to engage the communities around health and health insurance topics, and issued monthly press releases on health topics;
- Convened events and programs to address the health concerns that each community identified, such as health fairs, health screenings, and community exercise programs, in response to specific needs identified by community partners;
- Created and shared resources about health and health insurance, such as print materials, videos, and giveaways to raise awareness;
- Delivered health and health literacy trainings on topics such as health insurance for benefits personnel at small businesses in the community, employees at organizations in the community, and community members; and
- Provided dedicated contacts at Health Literacy Media who share free health resources with community partners.

Both large and small organizations, including health centers, school districts, community centers, and chambers of commerce, were partners in this effort. Healthy Schools Healthy Communities, a separate program supported by the Missouri Foundation for Health, was an important partner in Hannibal because it already had substantial resources in the community. This provided the opportunity to compare outcomes between low-resource and high-resource communities, explained O'Leary.

Discussing the key findings from the pilot programs, she said that community members in Hannibal reported a lack of community awareness about existing health resources even among health professionals, a lack of coordination of health and social services resources, and little knowledge about health insurance and the insurance marketplace. They also noted that health care organizations in Hannibal were using unclear materials, such as discharge instructions, and that there was a significant problem with mental health in the community, particularly among teenagers. One thing O'Leary's team did was to help the Hannibal community create a resource directory on a smartphone app called Johego to connect the community with the services it needs. At the time of the workshop, Hannibal was planning a community event that would bring together all of the community partners and the local newspapers to launch the app, and O'Leary's team was preparing to train providers and the public on how to use the app.

Another well-received activity in Hannibal, which responded to the community's food-related health issues, featured a cooking demonstration by one of the highest ranking female chefs in the U.S. Coast Guard. In addition to addressing a community need, this activity also introduced Hannibal's children to a non-traditional military path. "We talked about careers, but also provided cooking demonstrations and easy make-ahead meals," said O'Leary. "We gave them food and recipes, too, so they could go home and make these dishes."

O'Leary said that lessons learned during the first year of the Hannibal pilot included the observation that technology can help bridge barriers to creating a unified resource directory, that presentations such as the one by the U.S. Coast Guard chef can add value and exposure to existing programs, and that collaboration among community resources will improve the health of the community. O'Leary noted that the community has already asked for the second year of the pilot to include more information about mental health services, substance abuse, insurance coverage, obesity, and preventive health. The community, she said, is driving an agenda to which she and her colleagues are responding.

The residents of Monett, through a series of meetings with a variety of leaders and community members working in the health and wellness field, identified the issues they wanted the program to address. These included tobacco use, obesity and diabetes, cardiovascular disease, how to motivate the community to be more active, drug use and opioid addiction, and dental and vision services, particularly in the Latino population. One of the activities O'Leary and her colleagues created for Monett was to start a twice-monthly community walk, Monett on the Move, that included 20-, 30-, and 40-minute walks for people of different fitness levels. "We started with 4 people at the first walk, but by the end we were getting 40 people at every walk" O'Leary said.

Other activities involved connecting with the local farmer's market, setting up a health insurance booth to provide the community with information, and providing health insurance literacy training for the Monett school district and EFCO, one of the region's major employers. Face-to-face meetings and texting proved to be effective tools for building relationships in the community, and in that respect, proved important to finding social nodes in the community to learn about community norms and culture. Going forward, the pilot plans to target advertising to increase turnout of the Latino and Hmong (people from parts of Southeast Asia) communities for events such as Monett on the Move.

In Poplar Bluff, smoking, obesity, heart disease, drug abuse, and the high poverty rate were the community's main concerns, as were a lack of access to fresh fruits and vegetables, the struggle to recruit specialty physicians to the area, and a lack of transportation. Poplar Bluff residents were also distrustful of health insurance and the ACA. To address these issues, O'Leary and her colleagues worked with local partners to create a wellness fair that provided health, vision, and dental screenings, as well as health-related giveaways such as Fitbit fitness trackers. They also organized a trail run to raise money for an all-inclusive playground project and provided $20 vouchers to the farmers' market to every participant. The community partners, said O'Leary, have said that the issues they want to address in year two of the pilot include building the all-inclusive playground and trail connections and addressing tobacco, heroin, and prescription drug abuse in the community.

The big issues that stakeholders in Salem identified were food insecurity, poor nutrition, lack of physical activity, obesity, overuse of the emergency room for oral health issues, high rates of teenage pregnancy, smoking, heart disease, high rates of poverty, alcohol and drug abuse, lack of transportation, and lack of knowledge about health insurance. O'Leary said that the U.S. Coast Guard chef also made an appearance in Salem. Her demonstrations of how to cook healthy meals on a budget and prepare easy make-ahead meals were well received by the community. So, too, was a 3-day visit by the Smile Mobile, which provided dental services to 7 children and 20 adults and talked about avoiding overuse of the emergency room for dental services. O'Leary noted that this was the first visit to Salem by the Smile Mobile, but now it has a partnership with the Your Community health center. Free cooking classes, she added, proved to be a great benefit for both teenage and adult community members. One lesson learned from this community was that it will be better going forward for a small group of 4–6 community members, rather than a larger group of 15–20 individuals, to decide on the best use for grant funds in year two of the pilot.

One takeaway message for O'Leary was that communities are multilayered, with different gatekeepers for different groups in the community. Another lesson was the need for continuing conversations as projects and relationships evolve. Building sustainable relationships, she noted, takes time and respect. "One of the biggest things I've seen across the board is the need for flexibility as a core competency," said O'Leary. She also noted that the community has to drive the agenda and that the various partners do not always talk about key issues in the same way. "This idea of health literacy is important here," she said in closing. "We want to teach them our words because maybe those words have some power for them, but we do not have to start in that place."

HEALTH LITERACY IN HEAD START PROGRAMS[5]

For the past 27 years, Johnson & Johnson has provided funding to Ariella Herman and her collaborators to bring Head Start directors to the

[5] This section is based on the presentation by Ariella Herman, research director at the Johnson & Johnson Health Care Institute and senior lecturer on decisions, operations, and technology management at the University of California, Los Angeles, Anderson School of Management, and the statements are not endorsed or verified by the National Academies of Sciences, Engineering, and Medicine.

UCLA campus to receive management training. In 2000, she surveyed 600 of these directors, and they identified poor health literacy and poor attendance as obstacles to better health outcomes for the families they serve. In response, she and her collaborators founded the Health Care Institute (HCI) in 2001 with the mission of strengthening the managerial capacity of Head Start agencies so that they can provide health education and prevention programs that attract 80 percent of the families to outreach activities and provide culturally sensitive materials that family members can understand and use to take action to improve the health of their families.

Herman noted that her program has benefited from steady financial support from funders, including Johnson & Johnson, the Office of Head Start, the National Center for Early Childhood Health and Wellness, the Fidelity Charitable Fund, the State of Washington, the Kansas Head Start Program, and Pfizer. Another key to success has been the partnership that she and her team have developed with the national Head Start community. "They know we are on their side," she said. All told, Herman and her team have reached 140,000 families across the nation. They have conducted training in seven languages, primarily in Head Start and Early Head Start programs and most recently in other daycare settings. Their experiences over the past 17 years, she said, have provided a number of important lessons regarding the factors that make community-based health literacy more effective. The first lesson has been that business management tools are key to enabling Head Start agencies to successfully define goals, objectives, and an action plan, as well as gaining the commitment of leadership. It is important, she said, to give Head Start agencies the tools to engage staff, parents, and the community, and to provide them with low literacy, culturally sensitive materials written at the third or fourth grade levels. Flexibility is also important, because Head Start reaches so many different types of communities, each with its own culture and health needs, and data are key for continuous quality improvement. Above all, said Herman, it is important to establish an organizational culture based on L.O.V.E.—listening, observing, valuing, and encouraging. That slogan, she noted, was created by a Head Start director. "When it trickles down in the community, it really strengthens the impact," she said.

The strategic implementation model that Herman's team uses (see Figure 3-3) consists of multiple steps because as she put it, "no change happens without intention and without planned activities." The process starts with UCLA faculty and Head Start leaders training the trainers from Head Start agencies. "We share with them the tools on how to strategically implement health education and health promotion," said Herman. "They go back and then they train their families on different health topics." There are also reinforcement activities to make sure lessons from the trainings take hold and to keep the momentum going forward. This model is sustained by what

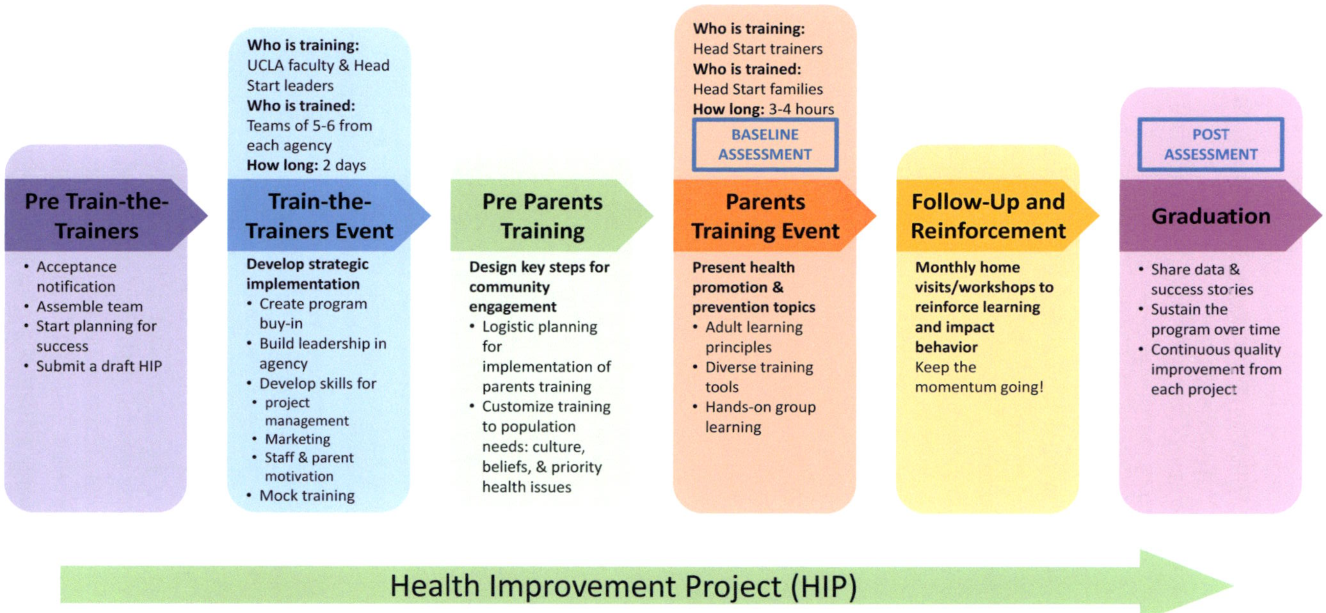

FIGURE 3-3 Health Care Institute's strategic implementation plan phases.
NOTE: HIP = Health Improvement Project; UCLA = University of California, Los Angeles.
SOURCE: Adapted from a presentation by Ariella Herman at the Community-Based Health Literacy Interventions workshop on July 19, 2017.

is known as the Health Improvement Project, an activity in which every Head Start agency must participate. It involves getting agency leadership to think about how they can engage their staff members so that they in turn will engage their families and the community. The Health Improvement Project also teaches agency leadership how to identify resources in their community, implement new programs, develop an action plan and budget, and collect data for evaluation purposes.

One of the training tools used with families is *What to Do When Your Child Gets Sick*, a book from the Institute for Healthcare Advancement. This book is available in multiple languages, and trainings of Head Start families are often conducted in multiple languages. "We are not trying to change tradition," said Herman. "We are trying to give understandable health tools to families so they can take action relative to the health of their children." Training is very hands-on, she noted, and aims to teach the core of what families of young children need to know, starting with common childhood illnesses.

Over time, HCI has developed a five-level evaluation process (see Figure 3-4). Level 2 evaluation, for example, uses surveys at the end of the train-the-trainer phase to assess staff knowledge. It also uses surveys and focus groups at the end of health literacy trainings to assess what parents have learned, and it administers both pre- and posttraining surveys to measure knowledge changes in staff and families. Level 3 evaluation assesses how the trainings affect behavior. In one study, parents were asked where they go first for help when their child is sick. Before training, 75 percent of parents said they would take their child to the doctor or emergency room, while after training nearly half said they would refer to a health book written at the third grade literacy level (Herman and Jackson, 2010). Similar behavioral changes occurred during pre- and posttraining on how to take a child's temperature and what to do when a child has a temperature of 99.5°F. Training, said Herman, produced a 29 percent drop in the average number of school days missed and a 42 percent drop in the average number of work days that a parent missed. Similarly, training reduced doctor visits by 42 percent and emergency department visits by 58 percent.

Qualitative assessment of outcomes for families and staff has shown that this program increases parental awareness of health warning signs, prompts parental response to early signs of illness, and leads parents to the appropriate use of health reference materials for first-line help. Families also report that they have a better understanding of common childhood illnesses, communicate better with health care providers, and make more effective use of health services. Herman's team has also found that training increases engagement of parents and staff in health decisions. "Working with Head Start communities, where it starts with pregnant moms and goes to parents of children ages 0–5, this is the perfect time to start engag-

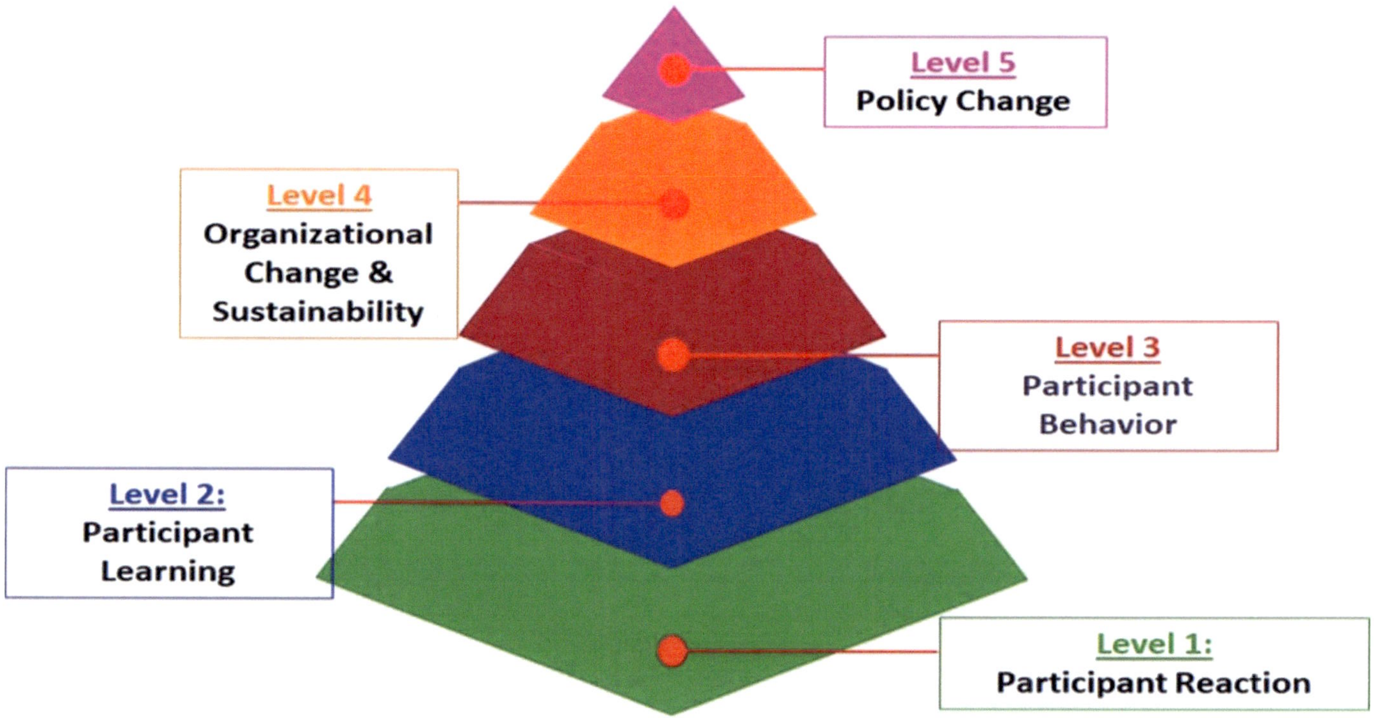

FIGURE 3-4 Health Care Institute's five levels of evaluation.
SOURCE: As presented by Ariella Herman at the Community-Based Health Literacy Interventions workshop on July 19, 2017.

ing families because they care about their children," said Herman. "When you give them the right tools, it definitely makes a difference." Quoting a letter she received, she said, "A parent who has the tools to make appropriate decisions about the health of their child has been given self-esteem. When a person has self-esteem, they can move a mountain," said Herman. "Mountains have been moved in the lives of the families that I work with through health education with L.O.V.E."

Herman's team has conducted Level 4 evaluations using long-term impact surveys of grantees they trained 5–10 years ago, well after their funding to implement the Health Improvement Project had ended, and found an increase in cross-sector collaboration within their communities. They also found that while the training focused on common childhood illnesses, many of the programs had adopted the model for a variety of health topics. With regard to sustainability, Herman and her collaborators surveyed 203 Head Start agencies from 50 states and found that 84 percent had sustained the Health Improvement Project activities beyond the initial year and 71 percent continued to provide this training annually without her team's help.

The key predictors to sustainable success, Herman noted, included engagement of the leadership of the Head Start community and the community in which the Head Start program operated, as well as providing incentives and removing barriers to attending training sessions. Many Head Start agencies have included funds in their training budgets to send teams to HCI so that staff turnover does not bring the program to a halt (Nelson et al., 2014). Nearly 70 percent of the grantees reported that they leverage community resources to sustain HCI training and 72 percent said that they have been able to continue providing incentives to parents as part of the training program. In addition, 89 percent of the grantees have adapted training to meet the needs and design of their local program, 82 percent were able to engage and motivate their leadership team to continue the training program, and 80 percent said that they have been able to engage and motivate staff to continue the trainings.

In 2017, Herman and her colleagues created a new online survey for both agency leadership and families that have participated in past trainings. The goal of the new survey was to identify the critical elements that foster strong, impactful health education and family engagement. "What grantees know is that once a family came to one training, they were standing in line to come to others," said Herman. "Every parent wanted this kind of information when it was given to them with respect and with materials that they can use and understand and that is adaptable to their needs." From the survey, her team found that the most important things agencies can do to continue to engage families were to first provide a meal—a meal means a great deal for these underserved families—and then deliver low-literacy messaging. Also important were rewarding parent participation in the interactive portions of training with prizes and having staff attend and mix socially with families.

With regard to which strategic elements of the HCI model were used by agency leadership to organize parent trainings, 74 percent reported that they used L.O.V.E., 85 percent used the Health Improvement Project activity, 75 percent relied on community engagement, 89 percent took advantage of parental motivation, and every grantee said that staff motivation was important. Herman said that the Health Improvement Project helps agencies repeat the training process in a strategic way. Every one of the 652 parents surveyed reported that they would recommend the training to a family member, friend, or neighbor, and 99 percent or more said that they were planning to use other health services in the community based on staff recommendations, that the training provided them with health information or other help that they needed for their children, and that the information presented during the training was easy to understand.

As she mentioned earlier, Herman and her colleagues found that once the method is understood and implemented, it is easily adapted with minimal investment to other health topics, including oral health, diabetes, obesity prevention, and prenatal care. As an example, she described the Eat Healthy, Stay Active model (see Figure 3-5) that trains staff, families, and children to have a stronger impact on both knowledge and behavior. Evaluation data showed that this program produces a significant increase in knowledge and behavior regarding healthy eating in both adults and children (see Figures 3-6 and 3-7). Perhaps most importantly, the percentage of children with a body mass index in the normal range increased from 59.8 to 65.2 percent and the percentage of children with a body mass index in the obese range fell from 30.4 to 20.5 percent when measured 9 months after training (Herman et al., 2012). She noted that at least one Head Start program created a farmers' market where children can learn how to buy food, and when they bring the food into the classroom, the children learn about calories and how to cut food and taste it, while also learning numbers and math.

Evaluations of policy change, Herman said, have documented changes at the system level in both Head Start grantees and the Office of Head Start Policies. Health literacy, for example, is now included in new Head Start performance standards released by the Department of Health and Human Services (see Figure 3-8). Health literacy has also been included as a crosscutting concept for the Office of Head Start's National Center for Early Childhood Health and Wellness, she noted.

With regard to her team's greatest successes, Herman noted that the HCI model strengthens management's capacity to better plan and implement health trainings; measure the impact of training on parents; meet multiple performance standards; use data to implement continuous quality

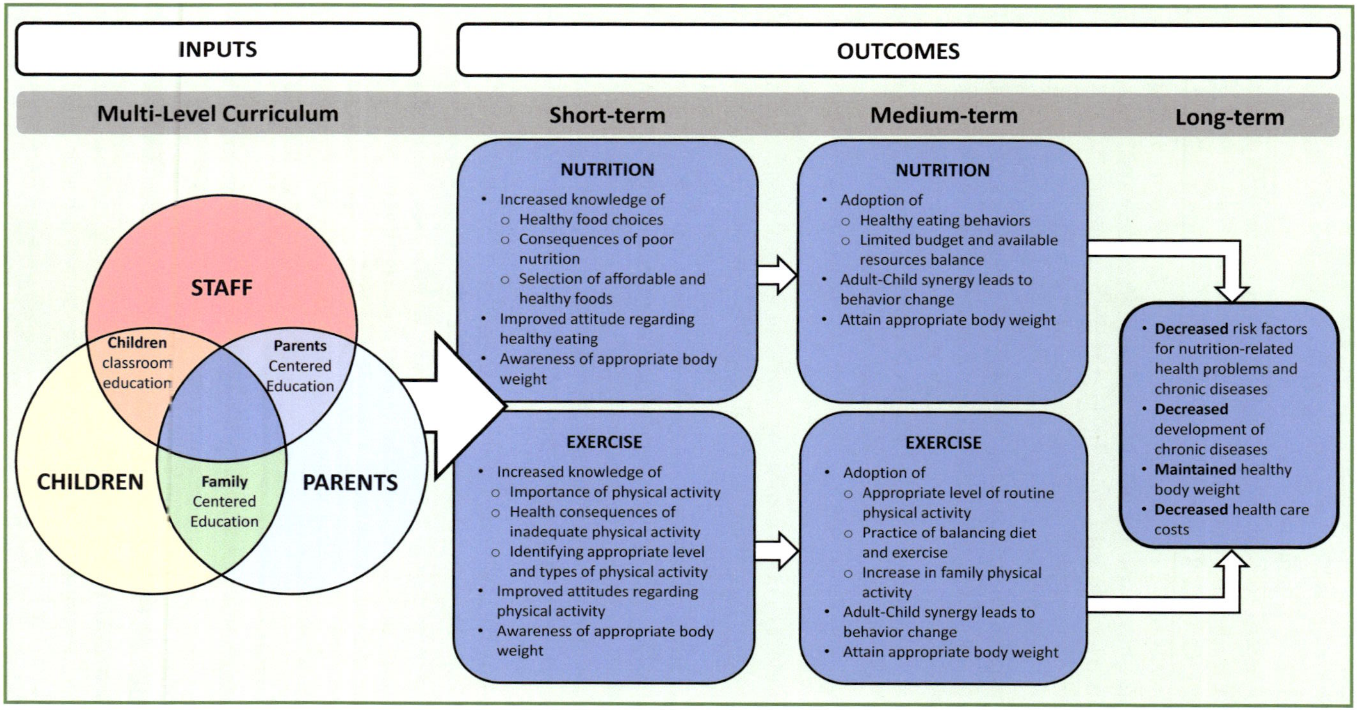

FIGURE 3-5 The Eat Healthy, Stay Active strategic implementation model.
SOURCE: Adapted from a presentation by Ariella Herman at the Community-Based Health Literacy Interventions workshop on July 19, 2017.

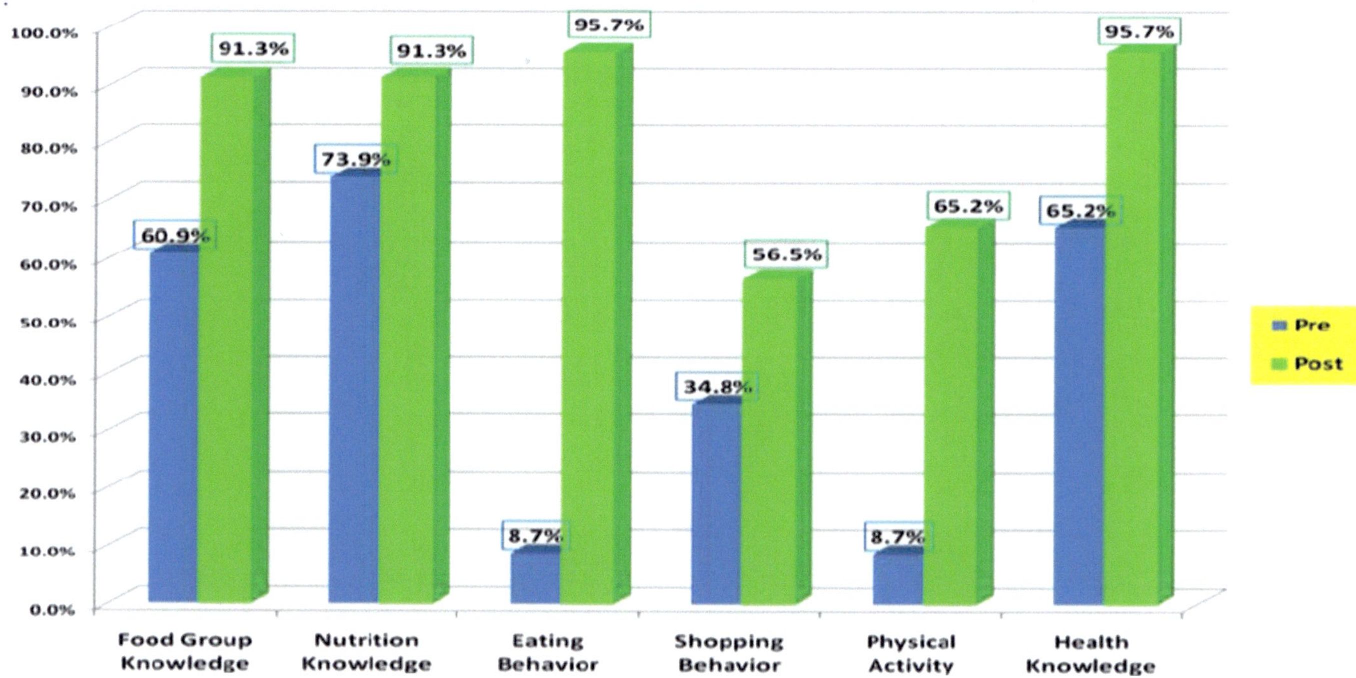

FIGURE 3-6 Sample outcomes for adults who participated in Eat Healthy, Stay Active pilot training.
NOTE: n = 497.
SOURCE: As presented by Ariella Herman at the Community-Based Health Literacy Interventions workshop on July 19, 2017.

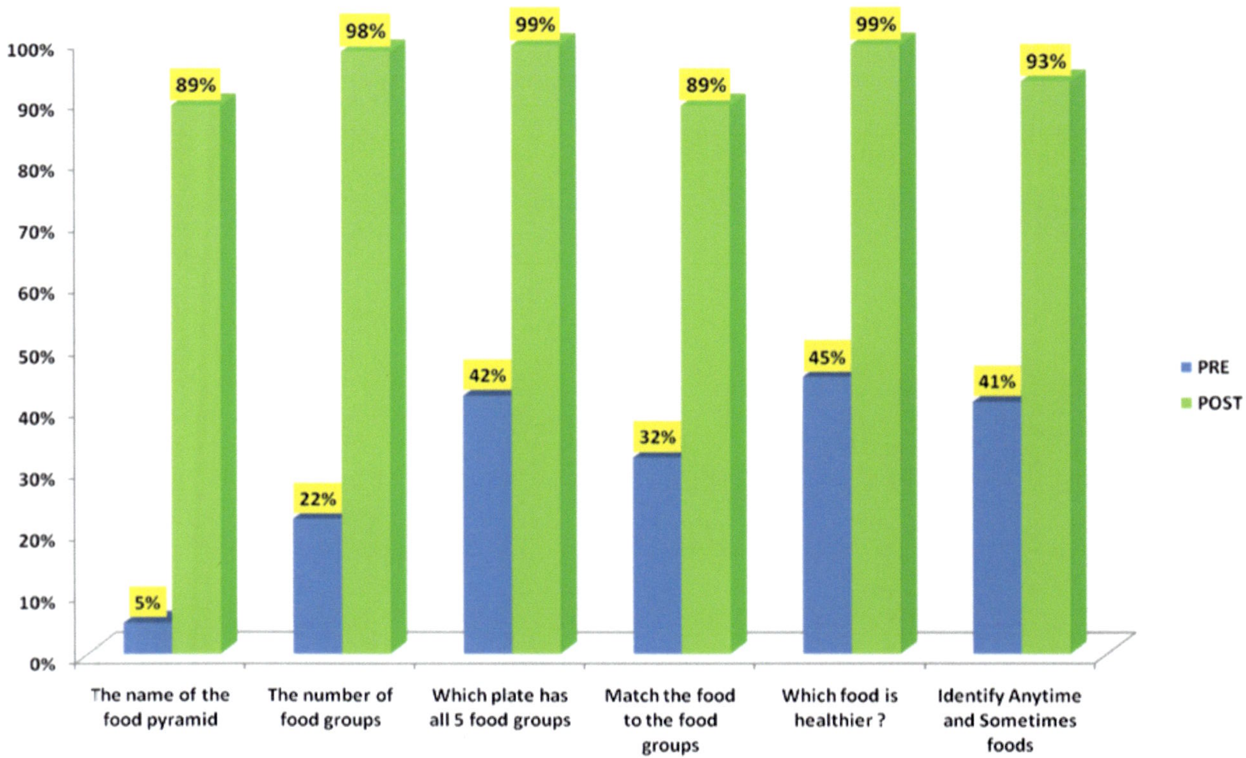

FIGURE 3-7 Sample outcomes for children who participated in Eat Healthy, Stay Active pilot training.
SOURCE: As presented by Ariella Herman at the Community-Based Health Literacy Interventions workshop on July 19, 2017.

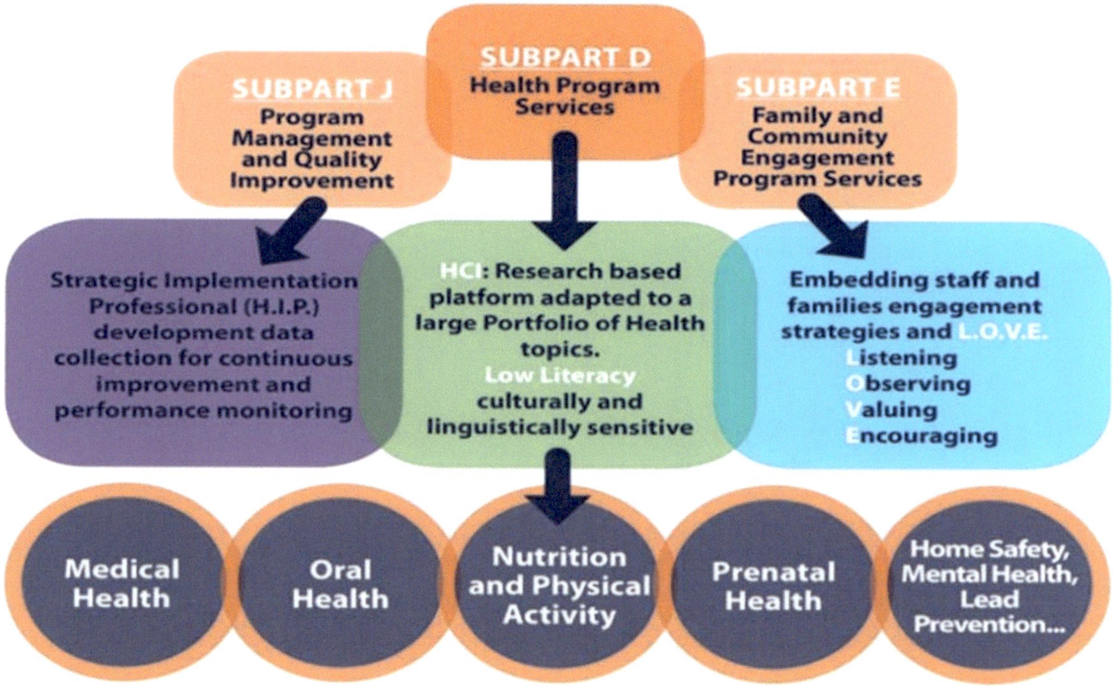

FIGURE 3-8 Many elements of the Health Care Institute's approach are integrated into the new Head Start program performance standards.
NOTE: H.I.P. = Health Improvement Project.
SOURCE: As presented by Ariella Herman at the Community-Based Health Literacy Interventions workshop on July 19, 2017.

improvement; build an internal culture of health and wellness; and enhance job satisfaction. The program has also strengthened community partnerships to collaborate on building a culture of health in the broader community, and it provides ready-to-use tool kits to equip communities to foster health and practice prevention. In addition, HCI's efforts have improved the health literacy of Head Start staff and families and increased staff, parent, and community engagement.

Finding funding for implementation has been one of the program's biggest challenges, as has explaining how all of the elements of the method are integrated, essential, and contribute to success. Herman said that she and her colleagues have learned that shortening the trainings, expecting less from trainees, not providing materials, or providing materials without training does not work as well. They have also learned how important building a team and building leadership are to success. One challenge going forward, said Herman, is figuring out how to embed this program in other settings, such as childcare and public school, that are heterogeneous and differently resourced. Other challenges going forward include determining how to take the next step to build parents' health advocacy in their own communities, how to ensure that the knowledge and experience of she and her collaborators at HCI can be transferred to an entity that can spread this work more broadly and continue to evolve it, and how to link this work with medical students, providers, and medical centers. Herman also pointed out that governmental and institutional policies will be critical for creating and sustaining demand and support for health literacy activities.

As her final message, Herman said that her team has seen that family engagement is fostered through health literacy and a management system approach. "Once parents have the knowledge, tools, and motivation to protect the health of their children, and barriers are removed, then meaningful change can occur," said Herman. "With a systematic approach to community-based health literacy interventions, we can make a difference. We can help set entire families and communities on a better health trajectory."

MODERATED PANEL DISCUSSION[6]

To start the discussion, Earnestine Willis asked the panelists to elaborate on how they set priorities for action when it comes to addressing the

[6] This section is based on the comments by Marisa New, board member of the Oklahoma Health Equity Network and chair of the Southwest Regional Health Equity Council; Leslie Gelders, health literacy coordinator at the Oklahoma Department of Libraries; Catina O'Leary, president and chief executive officer of Health Literacy Media; and Ariella Herman, research director at the Johnson & Johnson Health Care Institute and senior lecturer on decisions, operations, and technology management at the University of California, Los Angeles,

concerns of the different stakeholders in a community. O'Leary replied that her team used a consensus model process that first involves getting as much input as possible from community members and then discussing the resulting ideas. "What we tried to do is come to an agreement with the community about what makes sense now within a short period of time and what we can then do to get more funding to do more over time," explained O'Leary. Funding is not the only perspective, she added, given that many community partners have a limited amount of time that they can contribute to these activities. "We had to think about their bandwidth and what they could do now and what they want to do later," said O'Leary. She noted that as long as her team kept the conversation going and listened carefully to what the community members were saying, the list of priorities became clear rather quickly.

When Willis asked her if her priorities changed after receiving a community's input, O'Leary said that she comes from a background of community-engaged research and has the perspective that the priorities for action need to come from the community. "The strategies were not predefined for me," she said, adding that there are some things that she knows will work and she would like to provide those to the community, but the choice is up to them. She noted that she was never surprised by the priorities that communities chose given her experience that most communities are after the same things.

New and Gelders said that their organizations take the same basic approach as O'Leary. "We did not tell them what their priorities were, but we told them where to find the resources that would help guide them," said Gelders. She added that the Oklahoma Department of Libraries' only priorities have been to provide resources so that public libraries could become active, visible, and effective partners in health literacy, and to help Oklahoma children, adults, and families get additional resources and access to information to improve their health.

Willis then asked the panelists if they considered how to evaluate their programs and if they had adequate tools to do so. Herman, a statistician, said that evaluation is always on her mind, and when she and her colleagues started their project in 2001, they decided to create evaluation surveys on different prevention topics. However, when they went into communities to see how they were implementing their projects, they found that half of the families did not fill out the surveys because the literacy level was too high. As a result, what started as a seven-page survey is now one page. "We grew our evaluation method with the feedback from the agencies," she said. Herman added that every Head Start grantee received the survey data

---

Anderson School of Management, and the statements are not endorsed or verified by the National Academies of Sciences, Engineering, and Medicine.

from their community so they could learn from it. She also explained that her team has not used health literacy evaluation tools and instead created their own evaluations.

O'Leary said that her team also thought about evaluation at the start of its project, but there were no available evaluation tools that they could use off the shelf. "The communities were so different and diverse that we had to create our own," she said, adding that the availability of electronic tools such as Google forms and iPads enabled the team to create evaluation tools quickly and collect a great deal of data in real time in the four communities. One challenge the team faced was evaluating behavioral changes in the communities. "The question is whose behavior are we measuring when," she said, referring to the fact that behavioral changes extended beyond the individuals who participated directly in the intervention. "I think the tools are weak everywhere, but in community work it is hard to find a good tool that works for every sort of question and problem," said O'Leary. Her hope was that the workshop's session on evaluation would provide some guidance on tools that are robust and usable.

The organizations funding Gelders's project require evaluation, and every site involved in the project gets feedback from as many participants as possible. The sites then submit that information in the final project report. In addition, each site develops three measurable outcomes for their projects and reports on those outcomes. She said that there is always the opportunity and the need for new tools to evaluate these projects. New said that her coalition used the roundtable's 10 attributes of a health literate organization as the basis for the evaluation tools it has used.

The next request from Willis was for the panelists to speak to some of the strategies they used for transitioning from laying the groundwork to raising community awareness and building capacity in the communities related to their programs. New said that her coalition had just started building its capacity in its communities, which involves building the capacity of individuals who would be willing to volunteer their time to projects that improve health in their community. Within her organization, she had to find champions who would help take information about addressing health equity and administer a survey with the coalition members, and then provide trainings to those organizations. "That was critical in taking [the project] from awareness building to actually integrating it into our institutions," said New.

Gelders said that the first step for her project was to educate librarians about what health literacy means. An important service she provides is to be the person a librarian can call with questions, and to provide that service, she learned as much as possible about health literacy by going to a variety of conferences. "I did a lot of research so that I could provide some information and assistance to these grantees," said Gelders. She noted that her team holds regular conference calls for the grantees to share ideas, solve problems, and learn about best practices, and it also encourages them to share their successes at meetings such as the Oklahoma Library Association conference. Her team has presented at literacy conferences and at Oklahoma Health Equity Campaign meetings that are broadcast to most of the state's county health departments. She also provides opportunities for the grantees to receive continuing education in health literacy, including through an annual summit she organizes, and by providing funds for grantees to attend the Wisconsin Health Literacy summit.

Herman said that her program had the luxury of starting small, with 200 families, during the first 6 years of her project thanks to funding from Johnson & Johnson. They were also fortunate to have worked in the creative and innovative environment of the Head Start program. Each year, she and her team would observe the trainings, get feedback on challenges and successes, and then enrich the curriculum based on that feedback. By 2008, the program was being used in all 50 states and the District of Columbia, which allowed the program to receive an innovation grant from the Office of Head Start and enabled her and her colleagues to make teaching health literacy part of what Head Start agencies do when providing comprehensive services to families.

Next, Willis asked the panelists how they developed and sustained the resources to implement their interventions, particularly with regard to finding staff and volunteers. Gelders replied that her program received a grant from the Library Services and Technology Act funds awarded by the Institute of Museum and Library Services. These funds, she explained, are federal dollars given to state libraries to address priorities listed in that Act, and her program's health literacy projects address at least three of those priorities. Gelders noted that the project has received a budget increase every year that she has been involved with the project and her agency, allowing her to dedicate an increasing amount of time and effort to the project. As far as the grantees themselves are concerned, they use a mix of paid library staff, volunteers, and paid presenters. They also network with other health literacy programs in their communities. "They have been successful in getting in-kind and community support," said Gelders. She noted that many organizations are interested in health literacy, are looking for partners, and are willing to provide their services at no charge. She added that the Institute of Museum and Library Sciences is one of the agencies that the current administration has proposed eliminating.

New said that her coalition does not have any direct funding support, and it recently decided to become a nonprofit organization in the hopes that doing so will expedite its efforts to work with the Department of Libraries and other public and private institutions. In past years, the coalition sustained its efforts with in-kind contributions from volunteer partners and by working with entities whose interests lie beyond literacy, such as housing. "We are not talking specifically about health literacy, but [we] are talking about health and how we want to see health improved," said New. "Health literacy is key, but working with our non-traditional health partners has been one of the best things to leverage our resources and opportunities in Oklahoma."

Willis noted that when she surveyed other audiences interested in health literacy interventions in their communities, she heard that time is a scarce resource. Given that, she asked the panelists if it took longer to build their programs than they expected and if time was a critical issue. O'Leary said that her organization received funding in May and then spent the next 4 months explaining to the Missouri Foundation for Health exactly how they were going to use the funds and how they were going to brand their project. Once that process was behind them, O'Leary and her colleagues had to pick the communities and have the communities agree to be part of the project, which took another 6 months of work and regular conversations with the selected communities. Now that the projects are running, her team has found that time is an important consideration. "We are constantly trying to get people to have coffee or lunch with us because those are the minutes that they have," said O'Leary.

Herman said that she appreciated Willis's question given that she has had 15 years to work on her project and learn from the different Head Start communities across the nation. She said that although her program's resources were varied enough to satisfy the needs of those programs, the demand today is greater than what they can meet. She said that after about 6 years, Head Start agencies realized that her program exists to help them with their core missions and that the data her program shares with them can make a big difference to their activities. She noted that although her program has reached 140,000 families, they have 1 million more to reach. "We are not ready to retire," she said.

As her penultimate question to the panelists, Willis asked if there were successful initiatives that did not go as planned, and if so, if there were lessons learned during the development and implementation phases. Herman said that what she has learned is that there is no cutting corners. "When you do not do it intentionally, you will not have impact," she said. For example, some of her funders wondered why her program could not just distribute a book and measure impact or conduct training without distributing the book, but doing that did not produce the desired impact. O'Leary agreed completely with the need for activities to be planned and intentional, and added that once a program gets into the community, it has to be flexible enough to evolve with the community. "So many things do not go as planned, yet it all turns out okay as long as you are still there together," she said. One point O'Leary said that she should have mentioned in her presentation was about the importance of having humility, being humble and flexible, and recognizing that community members are the experts when it comes to identifying what their community needs.

Gelders said that her program has been highly successful and has had no failures. One outcome that she hoped was about to be successful will have been the direct result of her attending the workshop. To be at the workshop, she had to get permission from the cabinet secretary for out-of-state travel. As a result, the cabinet secretary requested a meeting with her to talk about health literacy and what she learned from attending the workshop. "I am hoping this will be another big success," said Gelders. New said that the Oklahoma Health Equity Campaign is changing what it is doing as it transitions to being a nonprofit organization. She believes that this change will expedite other changes happening in relation to health literacy as its primary determinant and to advance health equity.

Willis's last question for panelists was whether they share data with their stakeholders. O'Leary replied that sharing data is essential to helping the local programs make decisions about what they are going to do next. New said that program documents on a projector screen in real time, showing what people are saying at community forums, is something that participants appreciate. One reason for the coalition existing is to get comments from the public and provide them to city councils, Oklahoma Health Improvement Plan committees, and other stakeholders, she noted. Gelders replied that her program shares all of its data with its grantees. In addition, because her program receives federal funds, it must report statistics from each site as well as overviews and comments, all of which are publicly available.

DISCUSSION

Bernard Rosof opened the discussion by asking Herman if her program had any data on its effect on childhood immunization. Herman replied that those data are coming.

Cindy Brach from the Agency for Healthcare Research and Quality (AHRQ) asked O'Leary what criteria she used to decide which tools worked and what she did if a community had a need for which there was no evidence-based intervention. O'Leary replied that what works are the tools developed over several years of working with the Cover Missouri Coalition. She has learned from talking to assisters and navigators that many of the materials and resources that communities have are not accessible, and that her team can help with language and quality and get communities to expect materials to reach a higher standard. "We have data about what kinds of trainings and programs can help people change their knowledge, skills, and attitudes," she said. "We know that we can help people get to the point that they can make the best decision for themselves and their family. We have trainings to help people do that." In particular, she and her colleagues can deliver all of the materials that are the bread and butter of health literacy and have evidence to support their effectiveness. Her team has also developed a training menu for all of the program's community partners, and all of these trainings have been vetted and approved based on evidence and are available to the community. Her program has measures of satisfaction for some interventions, such as sending the program's public relations partner into communities to teach people how to do an interview with the media about health insurance, but the evidence is "looser."

As far as what she does when a community asks for something for which her program does not have an evidence-based solution, O'Leary said that she has 25 smart people who have the skills to find information, put it together in an accessible way using health literacy strategies for the appropriate audience, deliver it to the requesting community, and then solicit the community's feedback. "We do not make up messages, but get them from the evidence across the board," she said. For more difficult requests, she relies on the interns that her program gets from the graduate programs in the St. Louis area.

Paasche-Orlow asked New if she believes that health literacy is a social determinant of health. She replied that when she and her colleagues developed the position statement for their program, they looked at different sectors of the community and came to the conclusion that literacy was a foundational element connecting education and health. "Literacy is the determinant I am focusing on when I talk about health literacy," said New. Paasche-Orlow then commented that when states measure social determinants of health for purposes of risk adjustment in their Medicaid programs, they do not include health literacy as one of the items they measure. O'Leary replied that as a social worker, she would consider health literacy as not exactly a social determinant of health, but more of a crosscutting theme. Herman said that she would say that health literacy is a social determinant of health, but the problem is in how to measure it. Rosof commented that this may be the subject for a future roundtable workshop.

Terry Davis from the Louisiana State University Health Science Center in Shreveport asked Herman how she managed to create a one-page assessment that people can understand and respond to independently. Herman replied that it took 5 years and multiple rounds of developing surveys and getting feedback from focus groups to try to understand why they were not answering certain questions. Even then, difficulties arose when they translated the survey into other languages.

Andrew Pleasant from Health Literacy Media noted that each panelist has managed to "embrace the lovely messiness of community," and he asked them for any advice that they could provide to the states, cities, and neighborhoods that are trying to create coalitions and umbrella organizations. New said that her advice would be to get involved in a community beyond merely doing one's job by volunteering and being part of a civic organization or professional association. "Those that have been involved in our efforts have been those people who are the movers and shakers," she said. "Oftentimes, we say those are the same people at every table, but those are the people who are really doing things." One impact that she has seen recently is that those same people have started mentoring others to be involved in making things happen. "You have to go beyond just your work to share the message in many different ways that relate to those people you are encountering on a daily basis," said New.

Gardenier made a comment about the importance of paying attention to differences in perception and comprehensibility when sharing data with communities. She then asked how the Head Start project relates to the data Herman presented on emergency medicine and primary care. Head Start starts at pregnancy and serves children and families with children ages 0–5, said Herman, and she and her colleagues have learned over time that parents care for their children in the best way they can. When parents do not know if a child is too hot, they run to the emergency department, and when they do not know the difference between a teaspoon and a tablespoon, they can easily overdose a child and end up in the emergency department. "That is why we introduce hands-on tools over time, distributing thermometers and teaching them how to use them and what to do first instead of rushing to the emergency department," said Herman.

Wilma Alvarado-Little from Alvarado-Little Consulting, LLC asked if Herman knew of any partnerships that might be considering extending what her program has done with Head Start agencies to the elementary school setting. Herman replied that her program is trying to give families the confidence to understand and use health information, and she has not been able to track what happened to these families when their children moved on to public school. What she has seen, though, is that a large percentage of these families become part of the policy council and become strong advocates for children. "For us, it is a start at the moment when parents are most open to learn and to get the tools they need, but by no means do we provide a lifetime of tools," said Herman. Willis, who happens to be the chair of a Head Start board, said that many Head Start programs do have partnerships with school districts, and that with new performance standards, she believes there will be more tracking into the secondary school setting.

Lindsey Robinson from the American Dental Association thanked O'Leary and Herman for emphasizing oral health in their programs. She said that it is often an unmet need in many communities and is an important contributor to overuse of the emergency department. She then asked

Herman if her program has been able to measure its impact on families and communities as a whole. Herman said that her program's oral health prevention model is geared toward parents at the beginning of pregnancy and toward children, and she has not measured the community impact. "We did measure the impact in the community for our Eat Healthy, Stay Active model, where we measured the impact on families' knowledge, behavior, and weight, but also the families going into the community and making changes on what needs to happen and being much more active," said Herman.

Gem Daus from the Health Resources and Services Administration (HRSA) asked O'Leary if she has had the opportunity to observe communities acting on their own initiative to teach others and diffuse these innovations without the so-called experts in the room. O'Leary replied that because of the coalition's relationships, she and her colleagues have been in these communities for several years and have seen the resources they possess, but they have monitored what happens when the project team is not actively involved in the intervention. Herman commented that her program just completed a survey of Head Start programs and found that the thousand or so responding agencies all reported that they had become the center of information in their neighborhoods and are now going out into the community to give talks and discuss the resources they have. "That is, I believe, the first step toward expanding," said Herman.

Jay Duhig from AbbVie asked the panelists for their ideas on the greatest opportunity for using Web-based interventions to improve community-wide health literacy. O'Leary said that most of the issues that her communities raised had to do with eating, exercise, and moving, so while a Web-based program can provide information, the actual activity people need to do is best done with others. "Diet is not fun or exercise is not fun until you start to do it and make friends," she said. The opportunity she sees for Web-based programs is to provide information and facts and to build communities that connect people. Gelders said that this is where public libraries can play a role because they not only have the technology, but also spaces where people can gather and have the personal interaction that O'Leary mentioned.

The final question in this session came from Rudd, who asked the panelists to address the tension between the need to measure and gather baseline data and the pressure to take action. O'Leary said that tension always exists, and one challenge is putting the systems in place to make sure that any data that is collected gets reviewed and used. "Nobody wants to pay for that, and it is expensive and complicated," she said. New noted that it takes a great deal of time and effort to not only prepare a survey, but also to get it to the right person so that the response is meaningful. Herman said that her program does not experience that tension because of the partnerships it creates with the Head Start grantees. "They know that we are giving them the tools to be able to succeed, but as part of the contract, they know that they need to provide the data that we then analyze and share with them. It is a give and take on both sides," said Herman. "We are there for them if they have barriers, but they know that this is part of their responsibility to provide both qualitative and quantitative data, and they also see how we use it to make progress." Rosof added that anybody involved in quality and improvement work knows that tension. "It exists every day, but it should not arrest innovation," said Rosof.

4

Evaluating Community-Based Health Literacy Interventions

The workshop's third session featured a presentation on the issues and challenges in evaluating community-based health literacy interventions by Andrew Pleasant, senior advisor on Health Literacy Interventions, Research, and Evaluation at Health Literacy Media. Following that presentation, Cindy Brach, senior health policy researcher at AHRQ, moderated a discussion with three evaluators: Oscar Espinosa, senior associate at Community Science; Anil Thota, associate director for systematic review science at CDC; and Sherrie Flynt Wallington, assistant professor of oncology at the Georgetown University Medical Center's Lombardi Comprehensive Cancer Center (see Box 4-1). Brach used questions developed using input that the workshop planning committee solicited from people who registered for the workshop.

POTENTIAL ISSUES AND CHALLENGES IN EVALUATING COMMUNITY-BASED HEALTH LITERACY[1]

In Pleasant's opinion, ethical health literacy community programming requires looking at effectiveness and efficiency, addressing equity, and evaluating the program. Ethics, he said, refers to a set of principles of proper conduct based on a theory or belief system of moral values and effectiveness

[1] This section is based on the presentation by Andrew Pleasant, senior advisor on Health Literacy Interventions, Research, and Evaluation at Health Literacy Media, and the statements are not endorsed or verified by the National Academies of Sciences, Engineering, and Medicine.

BOX 4-1
Suggestions from Speakers for Evaluating Community-Based Health Literacy Interventions

- Remember that data about the community belongs to the people in the community and should be available to them in formats that are easy to understand (Espinosa, Pleasant, Thota).
- Engage the people in the community in evaluation efforts early and often (Espinosa, Pleasant, Thota, Wallington).
- Partner with other organizations or individuals within the community that have knowledge and expertise about the community (Espinosa, Pleasant, Wallington).
- Recognize that setting, population, and other context matter when evaluating a community-based intervention (Thota, Wallington).
- Build trust in the community by developing long-term relationships with community members and institutions (Espinosa, Pleasant, Thota, Wallington).

SOURCES: Adapted from presentations by Oscar Espinosa, Andrew Pleasant, Anil Thota, and Sherrie Flynt Wallington at the Community-Based Health Literacy Interventions workshop on July 19, 2017.

answers the question of whether a desired outcome occurred. Efficiency, which he said is rarely considered in relation to a health literacy program, is the ratio of effective output to the total input in any system, or the cost per unit of a desired outcome. Equity relates to the issues of fairness and justice and to the elimination of social, environmental, and health inequities, and evaluation is required to ensure that all of the above occurred and to advance the field. Pleasant said that he had found some beauty in the logic of combining all of these because being ethical requires being efficient, effective, and equitable, while proving effectiveness, efficiency, and equity requires evaluation. "Essentially, evaluation is an ethical approach to everything everybody in this room and in health literacy does," said Pleasant.

Evaluation has many possible goals (see Box 4-2), including providing evidence of success or failure, needing to justify a program to funders and management, and developing best practices and plans for program improvement. Regardless of the ultimate goals of an evaluation, in Pleasant's opinion the overarching purpose should be to produce valid and reliable evidence that can be used to make something better. In fact, said Pleasant, usability is an important aspect of good evaluation.

What evidence is not, said Pleasant, is a set of morals, casual conversations, a brainstorming session, continuing the status quo, or arguments in defense of past actions. Pleasant continued by saying that evidence is also not an opinion or value, a new idea that seems good, or something only a

BOX 4-2
Possible Goals for Evaluation

- Provide valid and reliable evidence of success or failure
- Justify the program to funders and management
- Document need for additional resources
- Indicate areas requiring program modification and improvement
- Inform policy
- Facilitate the sharing of best practices
- Increase an organization's understanding of individual programs
- Encourage cooperative ventures with other organizations
- Provide a basis for systematic reviews in the future
- Develop best steps and next steps!

SOURCE: Adapted from a presentation by Andrew Pleasant at the Community-Based Health Literacy Interventions workshop on July 19, 2017.

person with a Ph.D. can collect, even though many people treat evidence in that manner. One thing that differentiates his approach to evaluation, said Pleasant, is that he puts it firmly in the realm of research. "There are people who will argue strenuously that evaluation research and research are two different animals, and I could not disagree more," he said. "If evaluation does not live up to the definition of good research, then it is a bad evaluation. It is as simple as that."

In Pleasant's view an important yet often neglected piece of evaluation regards ownership of the data. "The data are not ours," said Pleasant. "They belong to the people who are fortunate enough to be able to work within a community. They let me use it, but it is their property." In his opinion, if he does not give evaluation data back to the community in a form they can use, he has not lived up to his part of the social contract. "If you do not think that social contract exists, then you better rethink your relationship to a community because it does," he added.

Pleasant presented a research impact framework that indicates areas of possible evaluation across all research and that, in his view, is absolutely relevant to health literacy (Kuruvilla et al., 2006). This framework focuses on research-related impacts, policy impacts, service impacts, and societal impacts. He noted that other frameworks are also effective, in that they help the evaluator to think through what to include in the evaluation metrics.

When designing a community-based health literacy intervention and accompanying evaluation framework, the number one rule is to engage community members early and often because they have the most to teach anyone developing or evaluating a program. "If you do engage people—

not patients, not participants, but people with names—you will naturally follow a path that means you are talking to them about their entire lives," said Pleasant. "You are not launching a program for people with type 2 diabetes. You are launching a program for people who happen to have type 2 diabetes and a whole bunch of other stuff going on in their lives that is going to get in the way of your intervention if you only focus on their type 2 diabetes, and do not talk to who they are in their entirety and do not include that entirety in your evaluation." The reason for that, he added, is that an evaluation will find people for whom the intervention did not work, and without addressing their whole lives, it will be impossible to know why it did not work.

Given that a major goal for addressing health literacy in communities is to prevent chronic disease, it is important to remember that prevention at large also means taking care of people who already have the disease. Prevention, said Pleasant, is not just about stopping disease from developing; it is also about reversing the course of disease and preventing the worst outcomes.

Following the simple logic of engaging people early and often, including their whole lives, and preventing chronic disease will lead to a robust level of health literacy, remarked Pleasant. Although these steps may not seem to be about evaluation, in Pleasant's view they are because engaging people early and often means conducting formative research and evaluation in a community, tailoring materials to meet the needs of community members, and engaging in participatory research and evaluation. Pleasant noted that including the whole lives of community members in an evaluation forces one to think about who to involve, when and where to ask questions, how and what to ask community members, and perhaps most importantly, who should ask the questions. In many of the communities where Pleasant works, "the last thing you want is a tall white guy with a pen and paper asking people questions, because that means trouble to many people in this world," he said. "If you do not embrace that reality and figure out who is the right person to be asking the questions then you are going to miss the boat because people are going to tell the tall white guy what they always tell the tall white guy."

Continuing with his discussion of the logic model, Pleasant said that thinking about prevention in evaluation terms reinforces the absolute need for an objective indicator in the evaluation. While satisfaction, understanding, and self-efficacy are terrific metrics, said Pleasant, those indicators cannot compare to measuring a drop in blood pressure or body mass index given that the goal is to help people create health in their lives. Regarding when to evaluate, Pleasant said that it is a mistake to wait to start an evaluation until the intervention is finished. The best practice, he said, is to conduct formative, baseline, and process evaluation, and to evaluate outcomes and sustainability.

Turning to an example of interventions that he has launched in communities over the past decade, Pleasant described the Life Enhancement Program. This integrative health program, offered in partnership with a local health care provider, covers all of the health determinants in a person's life over a minimum of 40 hours of contact time. The program includes one-on-one sessions, grocery store tours, group sessions, and hands-on practical exercises. The program, tailored to each community based on a formative evaluation, has at least 120 learning objectives. The logic model holds that improving health literacy will lead to behavioral changes. In turn this will improve individual health status, which in the aggregate will improve public health (see Figure 4-1).

In terms of evaluation, Pleasant said there are two approaches. One approach starts with the Calgary Charter's definition of health literacy (Coleman et al., 2009), which includes five steps: find, understand, evaluate, communicate, and use (see Figure 4-2). Communicate, said Pleasant, is incredibly important at the community level because communication—measured by how many people each participant has shared their messages with—turns into a diffusion of innovations. He noted that each participant, on average, shares information with 15 others in the community. What he has not done yet is to find those 15 people and ask if they shared their new knowledge with others. Self-efficacy, he explained, is a good surrogate for the evaluate phase because when people have gained confidence in their ability to act on their increased health knowledge, they have, in essence, evaluated themselves. Use, he said, is the indicator of behavioral changes, and participants in this program realized statistically significant improvements in blood pressure indicators, depression, stress, civic engagement, and other positive health behaviors.

The second approach to evaluation uses the Calgary Charter health literacy scale to assess the same five steps of find, understand, evaluate, communicate, and use (see Table 4-1). Using this approach also produces about the same results, said Pleasant. "People are self-reporting fairly accurately when you compare their self-reports to in fact a more 'objective' indicator of the steps of health literacy," said Pleasant. "You can do it both ways."

Theater for Health, another community-based health literacy intervention that Pleasant has launched, uses theater to change behaviors around health issues. The first launch, in Peru, focused on household hygiene and followed the process of identifying local partners, conducting formative research, and learning about the community. Pleasant and his collaborators conducted a 2-week workshop in Lima with the actors and scientists on the team to teach the actors about the science and the scientists about the art of acting so they could work together on stage. The program consisted

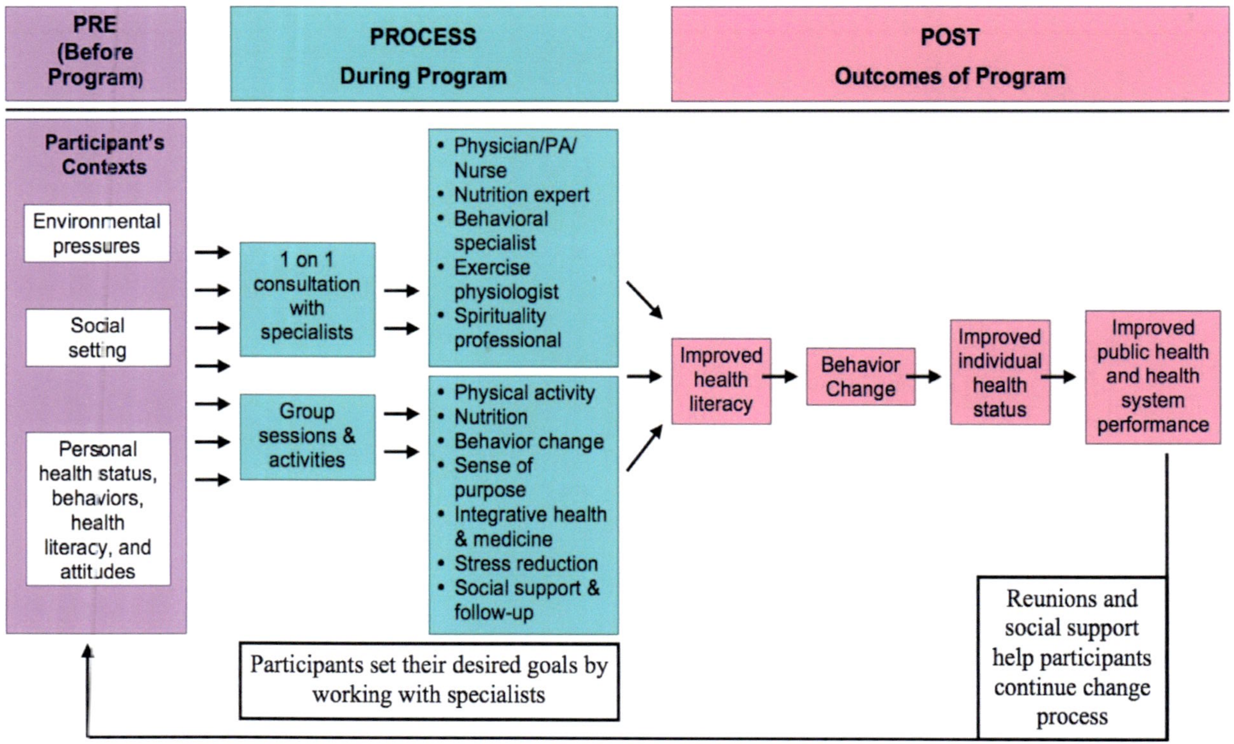

FIGURE 4-1 Logic model for the Life Enhancement Program.
NOTE: PA = physician's assistant.
SOURCE: As presented by Andrew Pleasant at the Community-Based Health Literacy Interventions workshop on July 19, 2017.

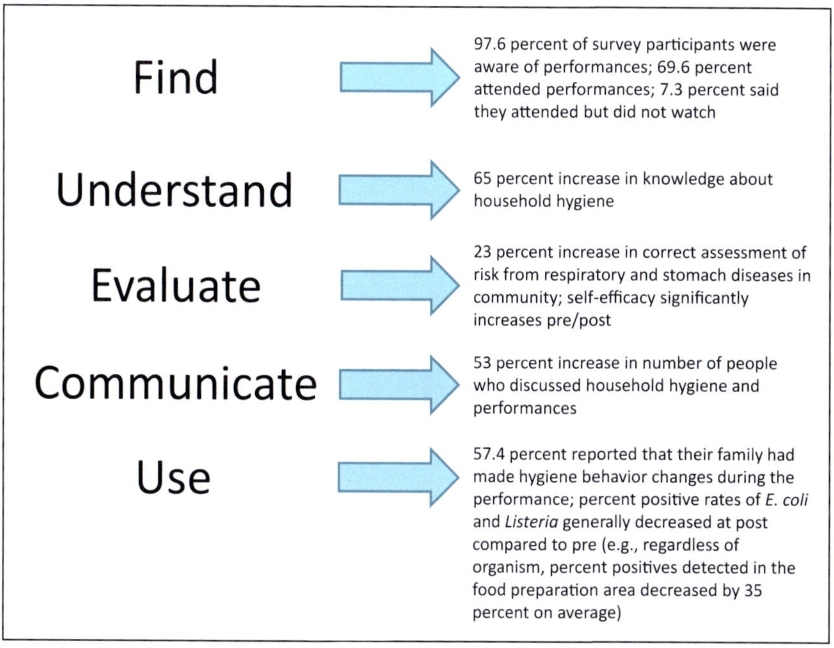

FIGURE 4-2 Health literacy improvements in the Life Enhancement Program.
SOURCE: Adapted from a presentation by Andrew Pleasant at the Community-Based Health Literacy Interventions workshop on July 19, 2017.

TABLE 4-1 Evaluation of the Life Enhancement Program Using the Calgary Charter Health Literacy Scale

Frequency of Engaging in the Following Tasks:	Pre Average	Post Average	Percent Difference
Find/look for health information	2.7	2.8	7%
Understand information about your health	2.9	3.2	9%
Evaluate how health information relates to your life (e.g., determine if and how information is relevant to your life)	2.8	3.1	10%
Communicate about your health to others	2.5	2.9	14%
Act on information about your health	2.7	3.1	14%

SOURCE: Adapted from a presentation by Andrew Pleasant at the Community-Based Health Literacy Interventions workshop on July 19, 2017.

of 12 episodes presented over 11 weeks, bookended by health festivals. Pleasant's team collected process data from 20 randomly selected participants after each episode, asking questions about what the participants thought about the performance, what they expected to happen the following week, and if they were going to start making changes in their lives. After the 12 episodes, Pleasant and his colleagues collected data from a random sample of the community. One difference between this evaluation and the one for the Life Enhancement Program was that there was no guarantee that the people surveyed after the performances had actually been to the performances, and in fact, some had not.

After a quick review of the Theater for Health's logic model (see Figure 4-3), Pleasant briefly discussed some of the evaluation data (see Figure 4-4). More than 97 percent of the randomly surveyed people in the community did go to the performances, though some 7 percent admitted that they did not pay attention. "That tells you they are telling the truth," he explained. "In your evaluation, it is nice to have some checkpoints like this because the tendency to tell an interviewer what they want is strong in human relationships." To build some internal validation into an evaluation, Pleasant suggested asking the same thing in two different ways to see if the responses are approximately the same. "If they are

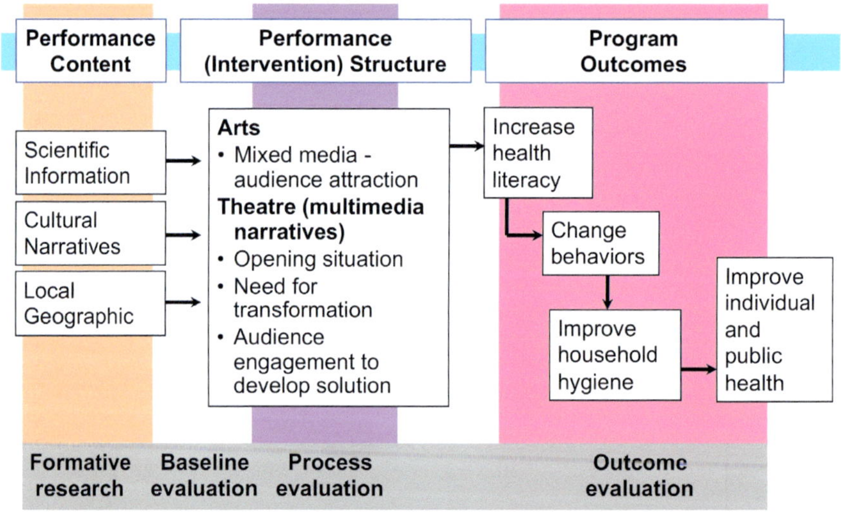

FIGURE 4-3 Logic model for the Theater for Health intervention in Peru.
SOURCE: As presented by Andrew Pleasant at the Community-Based Health Literacy Interventions workshop on July 19, 2017.

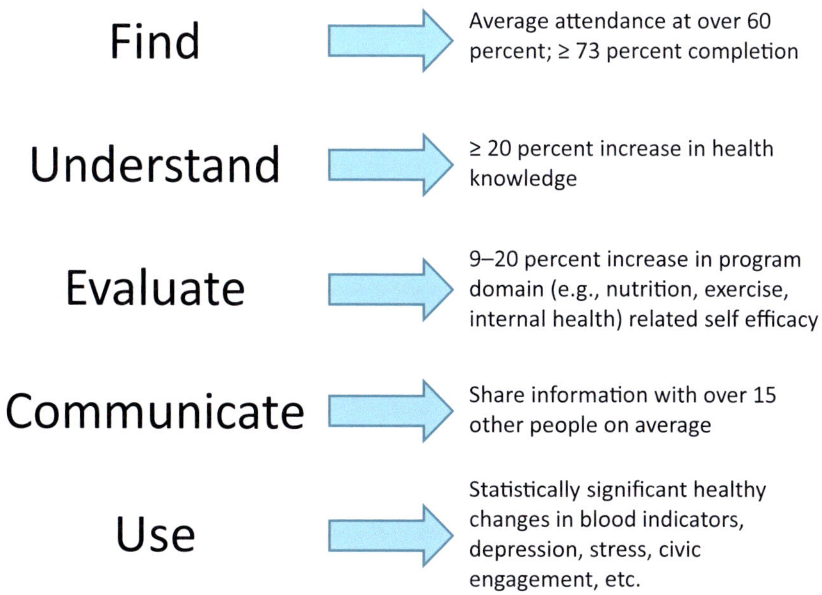

FIGURE 4-4 Health literacy improvements from the Theater for Health intervention in Peru.
SOURCE: Adapted from a presentation by Andrew Pleasant at the Community-Based Health Literacy Interventions workshop on July 19, 2017.

significantly different, then something is going on," he said. "It might be that people lied. It might be that they did not understand. It might be that your interviewer was poorly trained. There are many causes of that, but you need to check in on that." He noted that knowledge about household hygiene in the community, not just among those who attended the performances, increased by 65 percent, and more than half of those surveyed reported that their family had made hygiene behavior changes during the performances.

Pleasant's most recent intervention, the Healthy Table program, is a 17.5-hour program consisting of seven sessions with demonstrations on how to cook healthy food on a budget. Though he has not yet completed the evaluation, he has received reports that it is benefiting participants. "This is the smallest intervention, and we are still seeing that two people have reduced their hypertension medications because they reduced their salt intake," said Pleasant.

TABLE 4-2 Dose–Response Data for Three Health Literacy Interventions

	Dose: Contact hours	Response: During the last month, how many days were you prevented from doing normal activities because of physical problems or mental health?
Life Enhancement Program	40 minimum	41% decrease
Theater for Health	30 maximum	25% decrease
Healthy Table	~17.5	11% decrease

SOURCE: Adapted from a presentation by Andrew Pleasant at the Community-Based Health Literacy Interventions workshop on July 19, 2017.

The point of discussing these three programs, he said, is to raise the issue of dose–response, or how much intervention is enough. While all three interventions produced a significant decrease in one common metric—how many days over the past month a participant was prevented from doing normal activities because of physical problems or mental health—there was clearly a dose–response, with the biggest decrease associated with the most expensive and time-consuming intervention (see Table 4-2).

The message to funders is clear, said Pleasant. "Health literacy interventions can be expensive, but if they are evaluated well, they are worth it," he said. For example, for 100 Life Enhancement Program participants, the cost of improved health status in the first year following the intervention occurs at a cost between $376,400 and $570,500 less than other interventions to produce similar health gains. "This is what evaluation can and should teach us about what to do. It is not just outcomes or satisfaction, but how we change the health system and inform policy," said Pleasant in closing.

MODERATED PANEL DISCUSSION WITH EVALUATORS[2]

Given the fact that the randomized controlled trial (RCT) cannot be the gold standard for evaluating community health literacy interventions, Brach began the discussion by asking the panelists to discuss what they would consider to be the gold standard for such interventions and to provide an example of such an evaluation. Thota, commenting from the perspective of

[2] This section is based on the comments by Oscar Espinosa, senior associate at Community Science; Anil Thota, associate director for systematic review science at the Centers for Disease Control and Prevention; and Sherrie Flynt Wallington, assistant professor of oncology at the Georgetown University Medical Center's Lombardi Comprehensive Cancer Center, and the statements are not endorsed or verified by the National Academies of Sciences, Engineering, and Medicine.

someone who conducts systematic reviews, noted first that the RCT is, in many cases, not ethical when working in a community on a public health issue. As an example, he pointed out that it would be unethical to conduct an RCT to see if seatbelts save lives.

As far as a gold standard is concerned, Thota said that the Community Preventive Services Task Force, which has spent the past 20 years developing evaluation methods to use when an RCT is inappropriate, has put the whole concept of a gold standard on the back burner. "You think about methods. You think about transparency. You think about making everything very clear as to how it is that you did the synthesis," he said.

When his team looks at a study within the community guide review, they look at two aspects: the suitability of the study design itself to enable a sound decision based on the data it would generate, and the quality with which the investigators have executed their study. The study design, for example, might include a contemporaneous control group, which would be data from a comparable community over the same period as the intervention, or it may have a cross-sectional design. "Rather than say there is no evidence, we say this is the evidence we have," said Thota. For execution quality, he and his colleagues look at its internal validity and the epidemiological concepts involved, and the external validity, or how much the study contributes to the generalizability or applicability of the findings.

Wallington began her comments with a story about her first experience as an independent investigator with a National Cancer Institute Career Award. Her intention was to conduct a community-based RCT health communication intervention in select communities in Washington, DC, and to go beyond merely implementing the study to learning what the communities really think. She realized that conducting a neighborhood-level health literacy evaluation was not possible with the funding she had, so she started talking to people in the community to make connections and identify champions in the community. However, when she got into the communities in Southeast Washington, DC, particularly in Ward 8, where there are high rates of breast, cervical, and prostate cancer, she started hearing other priorities and had to adjust her plans to reflect those priorities.

In her opinion, there is a deficit of good exemplars of robust, community-level health literacy interventions, though there are examples of good program evaluation. Two of her favorites are the evaluations of the text4baby program and the Head Start program that Herman discussed in the previous session. Wallington said that she would like to see more mixed methods and multilevel study designs for community- and neighborhood-level interventions, and she applauded national funders such as the National Institutes of Health for emphasizing mixed methods research that combines qualitative and quantitative research. She also noted that journals are starting to publish qualitative studies.

Next, Brach asked the panelists for their ideas on some of the methods, data sources, and tools that investigators can use creatively to bring more rigor to the evaluation of community health literacy interventions. Espinosa, picking up on Pleasant's emphasis on execution as a key aspect of good evaluation, said that execution and engagement of the community will determine if a study is usable. One lesson he has learned from working in communities is to recruit people from within the community that are doing evaluation work or other types of research and make them part of the research team. "That is a key strategy," said Espinosa. "It increases the validity of your findings tremendously."

In terms of tools, Espinosa said that the key is good data collection and determining if the intervention led to actions that will eventually change health outcomes. Once again, he said, engaging community members is the key to getting quality data to demonstrate effectiveness at promoting better health outcomes. For example, when getting ready to conduct a pilot study, Espinosa has community members review the survey instrument to make sure it is something that people in that community would be willing to answer. "When you go into a community to do research to collect data, you are extracting something valuable from community members," said Espinosa. As far as specific validated instruments, he recommended looking at models such as the Kirkpatrick model for evaluating training programs (Kirkpatrick, 1959; Kirkpatrick and Kirkpatrick, 2016) that go beyond looking at satisfaction. This particular model, he explained, looks at four levels: Was training information delivered in an effective way to the participants? Did participants understand the information? Can they connect what they have learned to an action? What were the results of the training?

Thota's group looks at outcomes and study design, but also at applicability, and it brings in subject matter experts, preferably from the community, as often as possible to contribute to its study reviews. "We look at trying to get at the context setting, the populations, what is happening with equity, and what is happening with social economic status," he said. While that information is not always available, that is the framework with which he and his team move forward because even when the taskforces develop recommendations, people want to know if they will work in their communities. "Applicability is a step in that direction," said Thota. Above all, though, rigor is critical, both for the evaluation and the systematic review. "We map out everything that was done from A to Z," said Thota, with the goal of enabling people to look at the study and see if it applies to their specific situation or whether there is something they can do differently to make it germane to their communities. He added that the more context he can see in a study and the more context he and his colleagues can synthesize in the systematic reviews, the more useful it will be.

Wallington said that one of the things she has found most useful as a resource is the community advisory board that exists at most academic institutions. She then said that what most academics think of as community is not how communities envision themselves, and so it is important that community advisory boards not only include stakeholders from the health department, but also people who live in underserved communities and who know what works in their communities. She cautioned, however, that working with community advisory boards is a long-term process that involves investing in the community. "Communities have said, do not just call us when you have a grant due in 30 days and you need a letter of support," said Wallington.

One useful step that the Georgetown University Medical School community advisory board did was to create a community listserv that researchers such as herself can tap into when pretesting tools, for example. "When we need things pretested, we do cognitive interviews," she said. "We are not developing tools and taking these tools into the community and then having the community tell us this is not going to work." In one study designed to increase mammography screening among African Americans and Hispanics, Wallington and her colleagues developed a short one-page pre- and posttest instrument and training modules. When she pretested the instrument, some of the women did not know the word mammogram, so she had to redesign the instrument to use plain language and images to explain what a mammogram was without scaring the women by using words such as "smashing" and "pressing." After redesigning and retesting the instrument, her team sent the survey into the community and got a better than 85 percent response rate.

When Brach asked the panelists about the appropriate role for community engagement and if that differs for health literacy work as opposed to other community-based research, Espinosa said that he has been told by community members not to treat them like stepchildren. Engaging communities requires committing to a long-term relationship. "For true community engagement, it is all about execution," he said, referring to who gets invited to be on the community advisory board and who gets to chair it. Community, he said, is not just a zip code. "It is about relationships that individuals have with each other. That is what really creates a community," said Espinosa. One of his strategies is to recruit members of the evaluation team from the community benefit organizations working with the community of interest and the universities that are currently doing research there. That approach reduces the learning curve and it helps establish trust in the community, which he said is critical for measuring the intent of community members to act on the information delivered to them. "If they trust you, they are more likely to do what you are training them to do or what you are training them to help understand," said Espinosa. He noted that another reason to involve members of the community in the evaluation process is that it puts money into the community. "You are hiring somebody from the community, and putting dollars back into it gives you a lot of credibility," said Espinosa.

As an example of how to better involve the community in a project, Espinosa said that he has been working with a health care system that holds community health events in a parking lot at the hospital. His slight tweak was to suggest that the hospital should partner with an entity in the community, such as a church or community health center, and provide money for travel/lodging stipends for patients. "That made all the difference," he said. "It is those little decisions that you make throughout the evaluation that make a huge impact at the end and make the data usable."

Brach, highlighting what she had heard so far, said that the important role for the community is to help choose measures that will be meaningful to them, and she asked Wallington to comment on that. Wallington said that her first step in working with a community is to identify a liaison or champion in the community, which is usually someone who is well respected. In Southeast Washington, DC, for example, a woman named Miss Betty helps run a community garden and everybody in that community knows her. "You are not going to get anything done if it does not go through Miss Betty," said Wallington. "She is the eyes and ears of that community." It is with Miss Betty's help that she identifies people in the community who help her gain entry into the community, and working with her sends a signal to the community that Wallington is a person who the community can trust. "Communities have a good reason why they do not want to trust researchers or even participate in research," she said. "You cannot just walk into these communities."

Many communities across the United States are establishing boards that will vet research being done in the community, said Wallington, and going through those boards to get approval for a study is essential for success. The lay people on these boards will assess if a study will help the community and meet the priorities of the community, and it is critical for researchers to convince the board members that they are not there to do research about the community, but with the community. Her strategy before starting a study is to spend time there, going into the small businesses and getting to know the people, hiring a caterer from the community for the informational meetings she holds, and putting money into the community. Her team, for example, has hired two people from the public housing communities behind the Washington, DC, baseball stadium, and there is now a Lombardi Cancer Center research office in Southeast Washington, which is a medically underserved area. "When the community can see that you are actually investing and you are not doing what is referred to as helicopter research, where researchers come in, collect all these data, then run and write papers and get more funding, that is what helps you engage the community," said Wallington.

Brach then asked the panelists to comment on how researchers conducting evaluations of community health literacy interventions can ensure that individuals with limited health literacy benefit from the intervention, as opposed to just looking at the entire community. Thota said that when his group examines health equity in community guide reviews of early education interventions targeted to historically underserved populations, they look at applicability for specific populations in that setting and whether the researchers have stratified results by the different participants. Thota noted that as a result of listening to the workshop discussions, he will look closely at how to look at health literacy more explicitly in his group's reviews. "I think this group can help us think more about how we collect the data," he said.

Wallington, getting back to Brach's request, said that looking specifically at whether an intervention benefits those individuals with low health literacy has to be done intentionally, not haphazardly. It is important, she said, to establish a baseline that will help establish a target for those individuals. She said that she likes the Institute of Medicine's report on leading indicators for the *Healthy People 2020* initiative (IOM, 2011) as a source of benchmarks. At the individual level, possible metrics could be improved knowledge or adherence to a specific regimen. For example, in her work on human papilloma virus vaccinations, she looks at initial uptake and whether parents bring their child back for the second required dose. Formative data, cognitive interviews, and even motivational interviewing can be good resources for establishing criteria, metrics, and baseline measures, she said. Wallington also pointed to the importance of actually asking people if they believe the intervention is helping them.

Referring to the fact that some members of the workshop's audience come from underresourced organizations that are trying to do health literacy work, Brach asked the panelists for ideas on how those organizations can approach evaluation with limited resources or connect with qualified evaluators. "They are out there doing this work and want to produce the evidence," said Brach. Espinosa suggested identifying the community benefit organizations in those communities and seeing if they have evaluation capacity and to find those universities that are already working in the community. He also said that there are many volunteers who can be convinced to work on an evaluation project. As far as getting qualified and experienced evaluators, his go-to source is the American Evaluation Association,[3] which maintains a database of experienced evaluators, some of whom will occasionally work pro bono. Another strategy he uses is to break down an

[3] See http://www.eval.org (accessed August 17, 2017).

evaluation into pieces and identify who in the community might be able to help with specific pieces at no or minimal cost.

Wallington reiterated Pleasant's message that evaluation has to start at a project's planning stage. One of her mentors at Georgetown told her to always include evaluation in the budget of a grant. It may not get funded, but if it is not included then there is no chance of it being funded. Echoing Thota's suggestion to find the universities working in a community, Wallington noted that schools of nursing and psychology departments do great work and have graduate students who need projects. She also recommended contacting the Annie E. Casey Foundation,[4] which has started a national evaluation training program primarily for junior faculty and requires every Fellow who goes through the program to have a project to evaluate. "If you do not have a lot of funding, contact Annie E. Casey to see if your organization could be one of those project sites," said Wallington.

Another issue the attendees wanted the panel to address was how they can find out what evaluations have produced and how they can use those results. Thota said CDC's Community Guide website[5] has more than 250 recommendations based on reviews of community interventions that span the health spectrum. The website also includes methods and processes and contact information for the dissemination and implementation team, which provides technical consultations on implementation. He noted that the taskforce also identifies evidence gaps in its reviews, with the goal of spurring future evaluation research to fill those gaps.

Brach noted that the paper commissioned for this workshop can also serve as a resource. Wallington added that in the cancer area, the National Cancer Institute's Cancer Control P.L.A.N.E.T. portal[6] provides access to data and resources that can help planners, program staff, and researchers to design, implement, and evaluate evidence-based cancer control programs. It contains study protocols as well as promotional and evaluation tools, examples of pre- and posttest surveys, and trial designs.

Brach's final request to the panel was to talk about what happens if an evaluation shows that an intervention does not work. Espinosa replied that failure is very important. "I have certainly learned how to do better at engaging communities," he said, referring to lessons he has learned from failed projects. An evaluation can provide information on how to fine tune an intervention, such as redesigning materials so they are more understandable, changing the way information was presented, or rethinking the community engagement and recruitment strategies.

Thota seconded Espinosa's remarks and then expressed his frustra-

[4] See http://www.aecf.org (accessed August 17, 2017).

[5] See https://www.thecommunityguide.org (accessed August 17, 2017).

[6] See https://cancercontrolplanet.cancer.gov (accessed August 17, 2017).

tion about researchers not publishing what does not work. In his opinion, researchers doing good evaluations should not be afraid of failure because it will only make the next study better. Reporting what does not work also prevents others from repeating the same mistakes. Wallington agreed with Thota and called on journal editors to embrace publications that talk about what does not work in addition to what does work. She also said it is important when an intervention does not work to go back to the community and discuss the results with community members and get their feedback on why they think the intervention may have been unsuccessful.

DISCUSSION

Willis started the open discussion by noting that one of the key principles of community-based participatory research (CBPR) is equitable power sharing, and she asked the panelists, given the historical context of researchers coming into communities, how they go about power sharing in their work. As an example, she said that she tries to develop a balanced Memorandum of Understanding before starting a project.

Wallington replied that one of the most important aspects of CBPR and power sharing is transparency. She recounted one case where a community would not agree to work with her until she disclosed the salaries of everyone involved in the project, and her advisor agreed with that proviso. Another thing she does is include money for the community in her grant proposals, which reviewers seem to appreciate. These days, she said, many national funders are looking to see how grantees are vested in being equitable, and part of equitability is demonstrating that the communities benefit financially. She also includes community members as co-authors on publications, and noted that constructing community advisory boards made largely of community members is another way of demonstrating equitability. Wallington said one of the biggest compliments she received was when a community member called the main switchboard at Georgetown and asked for "Sherrie Wallington." When the operator asked if the caller meant Dr. Wallington, the caller replied, "No, she is just Sherrie to us." That, said Wallington, meant the community saw her as one of them. "When you can get to that point, I think that you are on the road to making sure that you can do this type of research in an equitable way," she said.

Alvarado-Little noted that some communities, such as an indigenous community from Oaxaca, Mexico, that she works with in upstate New York, do not fall under the community advisory board model and have a different hierarchy or power-sharing structure. She asked the panelists for their thoughts about how to conduct evaluations and include members from those types of communities at the beginning of the project. Wallington suggested that a town hall model might be appropriate for that type of community. Another approach she uses is to have a community liaison go into public housing communities to do peer-to-peer training and provide feedback on what people in the community feel will work for them. Espinosa said community health workers, particularly those associated with federally qualified health centers (FQHCs), can be a great resource. He suggested talking to them and providing a stipend for their time in exchange for knowledge about the community and the state of the community. Community health workers can also help recruit participants for studies, particularly individuals who may be hard to reach, such as recent immigrants who do not speak much English. Such approaches, he said, are particularly important when trying to reach individuals with the lowest literacy.

Paasche-Orlow asked the panelists how they use the term "community." Community, responded Thota, can be anything—people with a particular condition or a geopolitical community, for example. Espinosa said that when it comes to implementing interventions, researchers usually identify a community by zip code, but once they start to find out more about that community, they find that the defining element is more about relationships. "It is people that have something in common with somebody else," said Espinosa. For much of the work he does, community is the service population for a community health center, and even then, he turns to community health workers to define who should participate in an intervention. Wallington agreed with what Espinosa said about relationships and added that there are three important words that go along with relationships: sharing, equitability, and respect.

Brach, who comes from a cultural competence field as well as health literacy, said she thinks of communities in terms of ethnic communities and looks for the leaders of those communities. However, she said, there is often tension in such communities regarding who are the legitimate leaders. She asked the panelists if they had any advice regarding how to identify who those leaders or gatekeepers are. Wallington said the most important thing is to know the community, and that requires getting out of the office and going to where the people are. For example, she goes to health fairs, even though research says that health fairs are not very effective. The reason she goes is because that is where the community will be and that is where community members can see her and talk to her, which is how she starts building trust. "You may start with one person, but as people start to see you in the community, then other people will start to reveal themselves to you as key leaders in the community," Wallington explained.

Virginia Brown from University of Maryland Extensions commented that in her work with agriculturalists, financial educators, nutritionists, and horticulturalists, she has learned that the set of languages and tools are sometimes transferrable and that it is possible to borrow from other fields to make research and evaluation more impactful. She then asked the panelists if they could suggest tools and frameworks that health literacy researchers could borrow from other fields to enable reaching out to different communities. Wallington, a social scientist in the communication field, said that she and her colleagues have always borrowed from other fields, and one that she particularly respects and has learned valuable lessons from is medical anthropology. She also recommended looking at some of the models used in psychology research and combining them with tried and true frameworks such as the Health Belief model. The work she is doing now is based on a social–ecological model that looks at multilevel aspects of the problem she is studying.

Baur said that the Research, Effectiveness, Adoption, Implementation, and Maintenance (RE-AIM) framework and CDC best practices framework include valuable questions that researchers can use in health literacy work. As the practice section editor of the new journal *Health Literacy Research and Practice*, she encouraged everyone attending the workshop to consider writing up their community-based health literacy interventions and submitting them to the best practices section of the journal.

John asked the panelists where patients or community members who are not going to read peer-reviewed journals can find the results of an intervention. For example, there was a drop in the immunization rate in the Somali community in Minnesota that was triggered by an increase in the number of Somali children diagnosed with autism and the resulting barrage of misinformation from the antivaccination movement. John remarked that the valid research debunking the link between vaccination and autism is all in peer-reviewed journals, which nobody in that community was going to read, let alone understand. "Where do you suggest real information to the real public be presented?" asked John.

Thota said that whether an intervention works or not, there always needs to be some kind of translational mechanism in place to get the information back to the community in a form they can understand. Wallington said her group publishes what they call a lay health compendium, where they publish all of their research studies in a short booklet in lay language. Community liaisons then distribute the booklet to strategic places in the community, such as grocery stores, mom-and-pop shops, and schools. Her group also sends out a monthly newsletter; publishes short vignettes in ethnic, minority, and community newspapers; and uses a listserv to send out information to the public health community. She and her colleagues hold catered town meetings in the community at least two to three times per year, and her community advisory board has a standing meeting three times per year at which she talks about both results and future studies. She also holds conference calls if she needs to discuss something with the board. Within public housing communities, she explained, there are people who live onsite who can help disseminate information. Wallington noted that as a result of the strong relationship she has developed with her community, she often gets calls from the board or community members requesting help with a problem that may have nothing to do with her area of expertise, but she will connect the caller with a colleague who can help address the issue at hand.

5

Where Do We Go from Here?

The workshop's final panel engaged in a moderated dialogue that aimed to take the lessons from the preceding sessions and think about next steps in conducting community-based health literacy interventions. Michael Villaire, chief executive officer of the Institute for Healthcare Advancement, moderated the session. The panelists were Maureen Daniels, director of Berkshire Health System's Wellness at Work program; William Elwood, OppNet facilitator and health scientist administrator in the National Institutes of Health Office of Behavioral and Social Sciences Research; Michele Erikson, executive director of Wisconsin Health Literacy; and Caroline Young, executive director of NashvilleHealth.

MODERATED DIALOGUE[1]

Villaire opened the discussion by asking the panelists to comment on the challenges the field faces in creating and implementing effective community-based health literacy interventions and to suggest some possible solutions to those challenges. He acknowledged that funding and resources are the main challenges, and he hoped the panelists would address some of

[1] This section is based on the comments by Maureen Daniels, director of Wellness at Work at Berkshire Health Systems; William Elwood, OppNet facilitator and health scientist administrator at the National Institutes of Health's Office of Behavioral and Social Sciences Research; Michele Erikson, executive director of Wisconsin Health Literacy; and Caroline Young, executive director of NashvilleHealth, and the statements are not endorsed or verified by the National Academies of Sciences, Engineering, and Medicine.

the more subtle issues, such as trust, buy-in, integrating into the community, value, culture, language, and engagement.

Erikson responded that three things came to her mind, the first being the infrastructure of community-based organizations. Attracting and sustaining quality employees who are engaged in community work or who find the right balance between that engagement and not burning out from the work is a big challenge for community-based organizations. Health benefits, said Erikson, are sometimes a luxury for many of the community-based organizations she works with, and salary levels are often lower than what employees would make doing the same type of work at a for-profit institution. The second challenge she thought of was around buy-in and trust when working with communities. Wisconsin Health Literacy, she said, has been providing support, training, advocacy work, and capacity building for its members for 32 years. It has developed a strong, trusted relationship with its programs that enables the organization to understand what the communities it works with want and need, as opposed to the organization dictating what the community needs. Her third challenge was that of working in multilinguistic and multicultural environments. In one of her organization's interventions, for example, there were 35 to 40 people in a room, plus 6 translators who were translating at the same time and trying to make sure that the information was delivered in a way that was accessible and understandable for everyone in the room.

Daniels said that her organization, which has been doing outreach in the Berkshires for some 15 years, had an "A-ha!" moment a few years ago when it realized that it was doing outreach in the "hospital way," and not necessarily in a manner that truly connects with the community. "In the last few years, we have been looking at our verbiage and how we are approaching the conversation around health literacy," said Daniels. Instead of thinking about the health system's agenda, the conversation is now about the community's agenda. Her organization is also starting to be more creative with its solutions, using community health workers instead of nurses as a more sustainable model in the community, one that relies more on people who live in the community. Another challenge, said Daniels, is finding the right partners in the community who will be partners over the long term and who will follow best practices and use evidence-based models.

NashvilleHealth, said Young, is only 2 years old and is seeking to create a community dialogue and awareness about health in Nashville. Her efforts have centered around trying to bring groups to the table who have not been involved in health activities before, and that has involved a great deal of learning and understanding the many layers that exist in a community, particularly in the business community, she said. "As I learned, each layer has a different vocabulary related to health and medical issues, and there is a constant translation," said Young. One of her challenges is making sure that she and the people she speaks with are talking about the same thing and that they are truly understanding one another. As an example, she recounted a recent experience at a dinner for business women in health care in Nashville. As she was networking with the different groups who were talking about federal health care issues, one group mentioned payers, another talked about health plans, and a third was discussing third-party payers. "Now, I know that those are the same things, but does everybody else know that?" asked Young. "That was a clear example of the multitude of terms we use in this work." One rather simple solution to this challenge, she said, was to pick up the phone, call people, and have a one-on-one discussion with key members of the community.

Villaire then asked the panel for ideas on how the health literacy researchers can work with other organizations that are doing other kinds of work within the community that may not be operating under the same framework. An approach Erikson suggested is to help these other organizations become health literate themselves and to provide them with health literacy skill sets that they can also share with the community. Wisconsin Health Literacy, she said, helps train program directors to deliver health literacy skills to the community and provides them with information on how communities use the information they convey. The goal, she said, is for health literacy skills to remain in the community over the long term, not just when her organization is funding a project.

The issue of sustainability, scalability, and portability to other communities was the next topic Villaire asked the panel to address. Elwood replied that if a program applies for a National Institutes of Health grant, any standing, community-oriented study section is going to look for a process evaluation plan and set of deliverables that the community partners can use to sustain the program if it proves to be effective and if the organization believes it worthwhile to continue the intervention. In the case of Elwood's office, dissemination and implementation research have grown in importance, and it recently partnered with AcademyHealth to establish an annual conference and training institute to help current and emerging researchers learn the science of diffusing, tailoring, and scaling interventions.[2] For immediate action, Elwood recommended partnering with librarians to capitalize on their connections with community members and other community-based organizations who may promote health literacy without even knowing it. Another avenue for scaling is to act as a matchmaker among potential partners in the community who do good work and who can complement one another's efforts once they are introduced to each other. "When community members and community-based

[2] For more information, see http://www.academyhealth.org/events/site/10th-annual-conference-science-dissemination-and-implementation-health (accessed September 27, 2017).

organizations look to each other and give one another what they have, it is like stone soup," said Elwood. "They can provide better resources to more people or leverage those resources to reach greater populations than they do by themselves."

Erikson commented on the ability of programs such as Head Start to scale and spread its work thanks to the long-term commitment from the program's funders. Often, she said, funders have to move on to another issue, creating challenges for sustainability, spread, and scale. One way to address that challenge is to make sure that community-based partners have the capacity to report, measure, and evaluate their efforts and to provide the information so that program managers can make the case to funders that an intervention is effective and is worth continued funding. Erikson pointed out, though, that the community itself plays a role in sustainability and portability. "If the need is articulated from the community, the motivation to sustain an initiative is going to be so much greater," she said. At the same time, it is the responsibility of those who develop an intervention to provide the community with the tools and knowledge to sustain an intervention when the project's funding ends.

For Daniels, the key to sustainability is designing and evaluating a program so that it can be easily transferred into a community-based organization. "When you partner in that way, when you can get stakeholders in the community, whether they are in the business district, government system, or churches, you can have some sort of buy-in that brings different money to the table," said Daniels. That approach helps sustain an intervention because it becomes a community-driven effort.

Villaire's next question for the panel addressed the issue of how to identify partners for community-based health literacy practitioners. "When we talk about sustainability for subsequent funding for programs, do certain entities that could provide funding just want to be associated with some of these programs, and can we approach them for funding?" asked Villaire. "Do other entities have other associations or mandates or requirements for being in that community so that they want to be able to contribute?" Young replied that her organization, in fact, exists to form partnerships across the Nashville community, and she has had success when approaching potential partners with humility and openmindedness. For example, when she was trying to encourage the Nashville Chamber of Commerce to get involved in her organization's efforts, she explained that the health of the community is an economic development issue and that the community was not going to continue to be successful economically without healthy, productive workers. "It did not take long for that to ring home," said Young. "That was an example of us thinking strategically about partnership building."

Erikson recounted a story from her organization's communications specialist who is working on a dementia and Alzheimer's intervention. A board member from a literacy agency told her that pastors were working with patients with dementia and Alzheimer's, so she made a connection to the community pastors and established a training program for them. Other possible non-traditional partners she mentioned included seniors' organizations, homeless shelters, benefit counselors, and FQHCs. She noted that the American Library Association and ProLiteracy, an organization dedicated to increasing adult literacy, have created a national action plan to look at how libraries and adult education can work together on meeting the needs of adult learners.

Elwood commented on the Friendship Bench project in Zimbabwe, a country with 15.6 million people and 13 psychiatrists. This project has trained 300 Zimbabwean grandmothers in cognitive behavioral therapy and placed them on park benches or other open settings near health clinics (Chibanda, 2017; Chibanda et al., 2015). People arriving at the clinic who display signs of mental distress are told to go talk to the grandmothers, who actively listen and provide feedback and resources. "We are not seeing this just in the United States when it comes to community, but we are seeing solutions on another continent that we could use here," said Elwood. He said that one big step the field can take is for researchers, including those who do not define themselves as health literacy researchers, to actively seek out community-based organizations to partner together in order to advance the scientific knowledge of communities and address the fact that it is still unclear how people perceive health information and health problems.

The next issue Villaire asked the panelists to address was about how community-based health literacy practitioners can connect and partner with clinical health literacy efforts to produce better health outcomes. One potential place where such partnerships might work is at FQHCs, said Villaire. Daniels responded that her organization is a clinically-based health literacy program that is partnering with the community to implement the Life Enhancement Program that Pleasant discussed earlier in the workshop. The partnerships started with a formative research study conducted with the Canyon Ranch Institute and involved various community-based organizations. In fact, Berkshire Health Systems first tested the program on the leaders of these organizations, along with regular participants, and found that there were many issues with health literacy. "We keep talking about underserved areas, but there are many issues with health literacy with people who have bachelor's degrees and master's degrees who are smart people, but who are just not involved in their own health and well-being," said Daniels. In her opinion, it is important to keep that last observation in mind now that there are so many people who have high-deductible health insurance plans and no idea how to use them. "We have to keep in mind that health literacy is a concern for many people out there, not just the underserved," she said.

Erikson said that an important consideration is having the community and health care organizations identify priority needs together. She also said that it was important to find the synergy between what the health care organization is trying to accomplish and what the health literacy researcher can bring to the table. Erikson then suggested turning to the adult education community as potential partners.

In Elwood's opinion, every health, wellness, and literacy encounter should be seen as an individual opportunity to edify all three. For example, English-as-a-second-language instruction can serve as a vehicle for helping people gain health information, and cooking demonstrations can teach numeracy skills and provide health information. Similarly, the portals of most mid- to large-sized health care systems can provide access to tremendous health education curricula, Elwood added. He suggested that any organization that runs a health information site should look at the analytics to find out what type of information people are seeking. "That will tell you what your 21st-century community needs are," said Elwood. The community should also turn to search engine providers for the same type of information about community needs.

Villaire's last question had to do with champions, "Many times, we think of organizational champions, someone who clears the way for policies and procedures, but that is a very narrow definition," said Villaire. "Within a community-based intervention, champions are those people who are really embedded in the community or those who kind of help us to get into there." The question, he asked, is, "How do we identify champions or the role of a champion? Can we groom a champion?"

Daniels said her program has both kind of champions. Her chief executive officer is the champion for policy and procedure changes, she said. In response to finding out that he had type 2 diabetes, he came to understand the wellness component of health and moved the organization to adopt a more integrative health model. Within the community, she said, champions came to fore quickly when working with the Life Enhancement Program. "They wanted to share their story and talk about it," she said. "They wanted to go back to work and talk about it in break rooms." One participant, she said, went on to become a certified wellness coach and got a job working in the community on health literacy. "I think there is plenty of opportunity for champions as long as they are given the opportunity to rise," said Daniels.

Young said that NashvilleHealth has benefited from having former Senator William Frist (R-TN), a heart surgeon with deep roots in the community, as its champion. "He really served to catalyze the community," she said, adding that she does not think every group has to have a champion of that stature. "It is just someone who is credible, approachable, and who knows the issue."

DISCUSSION

Rosof opened the discussion by asking the panelists how they assess resources and identify trusted community partners who want to improve community health or be truly involved in the community when a health care system's service area encompasses multiple zip codes. Erikson replied that there must be a level of passion and interest in the community, which means that health care organizations should look for champions who are already integrated into the community. "You know it is a good fit if you can already tell their level of investment," said Erikson. "In those initial conversations about engaging with partners, you get a sense right from the get-go whether or not this is coming from a place of deep concern, commitment, and passion or whether it is coming from a need to check a box. If it is a need to check a box, then I do not think they are your partner."

Daniels said that she relies on her hospital's community advisory committee, which reviews all of the health system's community outreach programming and comprises stakeholders from a variety of different community venues. She also refers to the county health rankings to help steer the conversation of what the health system needs to work on to change. Villaire added that an obvious thing to look at regarding resources is to identify who in the community is currently responsible for disseminating health information. As an example, the family resource center that his organization runs in north Orange County, California, a medically underserved area, provides access to community resources for individuals who come to the center. Contacting the center would therefore be a good starting point for a health system that wants to identify and connect with community resources. His organization's center has already mobilized the community and organized the community's resources to provide services to the community. "To the extent that your community is already engaged, at a minimum you are going to have one of these social services agencies like a family resource center," said Villaire.

That is, in fact, what the system with which he is affiliated, Northwell Health, has done, said Rosof. "We went to our family health center, right to the community that probably needs it the most, and posted on various walls and had the entry nurses ask if people would like to be on the community advisory board," he explained. This approach, he said, has been very successful and enabled the health system to identify individuals who likely never would have become involved otherwise.

Dillaha commented that some of the champions might be policy makers who are not members of the community, but whose constituents live in the community, and she asked the panelists for ideas on how to leverage the input that community members can give to those policy makers. Young replied that her organization has, in fact, invited local and state policy makers to be on various working groups, and some of them have participated in those groups. NashvilleHealth has also supported legislation related to those working groups. Villaire agreed that legislators and other policy makers need to be brought in as part of any effort to bring as broad a spectrum as possible to the table. An important point to remember, though, is to get policy makers involved as early as possible and not wait until a policy recommendation is ready.

Baur commented on the fact that 9 out of 10 Americans have limited health literacy and that today's efforts to improve on that statistic are not making progress fast enough. As an example, she noted that the Head Start program that Herman discussed, as successful as it is, has reached only 140,000 families out of 1 million. "We really have to grapple with scale, and we saw that in the review we did," said Baur. Daniels replied that she was concerned about the scale issue when thinking about how the Life Enhancement Program only reached 20 people over the 12-week program, but when the sharing data came in, they showed that the program's effect went well beyond those 20 people. One radio show host, for example, shared what she was learning from the program on her show every morning and told Daniels's team that callers to her show talked about the program with her every morning. She also noted that spouses of people who went through the program started losing weight because of the behavioral changes that their spouses were making. "Scalability is an issue and can be overwhelming until you bring it down to who you helped today," said Daniels.

Erikson remarked that people in the community are not the only ones who need better health literacy skills; those working in the health care field also need to improve their skills. She applauded the ongoing accreditation and certification in health literacy initiative because she believes that embedding health literacy principles in the DNA of everyone coming into the health care field can help reach scalability efficiently. Elwood added that more research is needed on the cognitive and biological processes involved in the exposure to, perception of, and processing of health information to make health care decisions in order to increase the knowledge base on how to best disseminate evidence-based interventions on a large scale. Rosof said that he likes the idea of creating a learning health system around the issue of scale, which could reduce the time from discovery to scale and spread. Baur commented that she would like to see the sponsors of an innovation, when thinking about partners, to find those partners who are working at a bigger scale, such as statewide associations, and to test interventions on a bigger scale by involving those partners who are used to thinking on a bigger scale themselves. One added benefit of such an approach is that it would likely provide a better pitch to policy makers.

Baur also commented on the importance of including the community in the science of health literacy and helping community members grasp the scientific method, and she worried that researchers are largely keeping the science to themselves. Elwood disagreed, saying that "when you are teaching people about healthier eating or managing their blood pressure or glucose levels, you are teaching science to all of those people. They may not realize or perceive it as learning health science, but they are." His point was that when someone learns to tell the difference between a teaspoon and tablespoon, they can transfer that knowledge to other parts of their lives. Baur explained that the reason she brought up science is that she and her colleagues found it difficult to compare the different interventions they identified in their literature review. In her opinion, too much of the science in publications is a black box, particularly with regard to what behaviors or processes an intervention changes in individuals and communities. Erikson said that her experience with establishing academic partnerships for community-based interventions is that Institutional Review Boards can create barriers to publishing work in the community.

Pleasant asked the panelists to talk about the incentives that they have found useful when working with various audiences to build support in the community. Erikson said that Wisconsin Health Literacy incentivizes community members to participate in its patient advisory councils and attend the meetings with cash and food. She added that a less tangible but highly valued incentive of participating in an advisory council is the ability to meet people, form new friendships, and find new partners and identify new resources in the community for their organizations. The other side of that incentive, noted Villaire, is that organizations get to explain what they do to the other members of an advisory group or working group and advance their particular missions with a community in the context of the group's efforts. He added that one of his organization's community partners is an organic grocery store that gives away fresh produce at every community event, be it a back-to-school fair, a senior fair, or a wellness fair, which helps increase turnout at these events.

Parker asked Young to address how she speaks about health literacy as an economic driver when she talks to the business community. Young replied that Nashville's business community is interesting because it is a headquarters town for many national health care companies. These companies generate some $80 billion in annual revenues and together are the largest employer in the community. She noted, though, that it was challenging to bridge the gap between the health care business world and the community health care world. Her advice was to be very deliberate in conversations with the business community, talk specifically about the social determinants of health, and to use data to remind them about the scope of any health care issues, including health literacy. She cites data, for example, showing that the infant mortality rate in the community is on par with that of Libya and Russia, and she then describes how that impacts the future economic growth of the community.

Robert Logan from the National Library of Medicine commented that he does not believe the scaling issue to be as big of an issue as many believe thanks to the concept of innovation diffusion. This concept holds that getting to opinion leaders, rather than early adopters, leads to the most rapid diffusion of innovation and facilitates an easier process for strategic planning. "I think it makes it more possible to say we will never reach 90 percent of the population, but if you reach certain opinion leaders in certain kinds of communities and have an organized way of doing that over time, you will reach a good percentage of the population," said Logan. To illustrate the point, he noted how quickly American society has adopted all kinds of health and technology innovations over the past 50 years. In Paasche-Orlow's opinion, creating a tool kit for community-based organizations that explains how to engage in health literacy work and assess current organizational attributes as they relate to health literacy would accelerate scaling.

Steven Rush from UnitedHealth Group said that he is not sure there is a difference between rolling out health literacy within a community and within an organization. "There is a level of diversity and equity in both," he said. He also pointed to the importance of talking to specific partners in their language. "When you talk with the Chamber of Commerce, you use Chamber of Commerce language," said Rush. "We have talked today about the concept of speaking to people where they are at the time they are at." He also suggested that the field is about to reach a tipping point with respect to scaling health literacy interventions.

Rosof concluded the discussion with a story about Donald Berwick, former administrator of the Centers for Medicare & Medicaid Services, who when addressing his daughter's medical school graduation class told the newly minted health care professionals to take off their white coats and stand among their patients, friends, and peers and just listen to them. "When I think about that, I often think about trusted people and the importance of what we are trying to say and stand among those who need you most and listen," said Rosof.

6

Reflections on the Day[1]

In keeping with the roundtable's traditional practice, the workshop ended with each member reflecting on the day's presentations and discussions. Daus said that the message he heard was on the importance of listening, observing, valuing, and encouraging, which he said translates into showing love for your community, whatever community means in a particular context. He also heard people talk about "doing with" rather than "doing to" the community. His final comment was how sobering it was to see that so many of the studies included in the commissioned review paper had small sample sizes and could not quantify what they were able to accomplish.

Dillaha agreed with Daus on the importance of linking good community health literacy interventions with love and respect for the community, and to do so with humility. She also noted the need for public health organizations at all levels to fund people who can spend their time developing and sustaining trusted relationships. "To me, that is something that has not been part of the organizational or funding structure, and we really need that," said Dillaha.

As someone who works within communities, Willis said that she realizes that defining community is a continuous struggle, and how important it is to recognize that the definition of any community is contextual and evolving. She noted that the social and economic models in use have to be

[1] This section is based on the comments of the Roundtable on Health Literacy members who were present at the workshop, and the statements are not endorsed or verified by the National Academies of Sciences, Engineering, and Medicine.

more sophisticated and complex, and that the health literacy community needs to develop more tools to work with these complex communities. With regard to the key messages she heard, Willis said that the presentations and discussions consistently articulated the need to include more voices in the community in partnerships with researchers as a means of broadening the field's horizons of where more rigor is needed when it comes to the science. She also said that it sounds as though researchers still need to pay more attention to not taking models and superimposing them on the community.

Rudd said that she liked the combination of starting with a rigorous academic perspective on this work and following up with a concrete and innovative community-based program. She was concerned, however, that nobody was talking about community-based health education, a field for which there is a rigorous, evidence-based foundation developed from the 1950s through the 1980s. She noted that many of the challenges mentioned throughout the day have counterparts in fields such as anthropology and sociology, which documented the activities and engagements of communities in the civil rights movement, the HIV/AIDS epidemic response, and the women's health movement. "Many of the dilemmas that were raised today have answers that are well documented and well researched," said Rudd.

Commenting from the view of someone who has done community interventions in a number of fields for 20 years, O'Leary agreed with Rudd that it is important to look at solutions developed by other fields and consider how to apply the lessons those programs have accumulated to designing, implementing, and scaling health literacy interventions. She commented, though, that the day's discussions made her realize that the field is making progress, and though it may seem slow, progress is happening as communities develop their resources, learn how to fit them together, and bring communities to a place where they want to change. In her opinion, the table is big enough for everybody to participate, and community interventions need to bring in people who are just waiting to be asked to participate.

Terri Ann Parnell from Health Literacy Partners said that the key concepts she heard over the course of the day were the importance of innovation, flexibility, building relationships, creativity, and trust. These take time to develop, she said, and developing them is hard work. "I think sometimes we want a quick fix or the magic wand," said Parnell. "That is not the way to have sustainable, scalable change." Given the amount of work being done in the area of community-based health literacy, she believes that steady progress, breaking down silos, and working together on large-scale initiatives can truly make a difference.

Kim Parson from Humana said that she believes that the systems and structures exist to scale up health literacy interventions, but that the field is not leveraging them as it should. She also noted that payers need to be at the table together with librarians and school systems, and that by taking advantage of each partner's strengths, the field will get to where it wants to be much faster. Alvarado-Little stressed the importance of involving public libraries as partners in community health literacy interventions.

Amanda Wilson from the National Library of Medicine reiterated the message that libraries are willing partners and the health literacy field should reach out more to the library community. Libraries, she said, are part of a system that can help support scale, particularly at the level of city- and county-wide implementation. She noted that National Network of Libraries of Medicine members receive funding to have time for relationship building and they have been doing so in their communities for many years. This network, she said, is looking at ways of partnering with the Public Library Association and the American Library Association on work addressing health and wellness questions that come to their libraries. As a final thought, she said that the important words she heard throughout the day included humility, flexibility, and love.

Rush said that one of the messages he heard was about the importance of collaborative thinking involving those who are developing health literacy interventions and those who live in the community, with the community teaching the developers about its culture, its needs, its issues, and its concerns. Collaborative thinking will lead to understanding, trust, and buy-in. "If people do not trust, they are going to have difficulty making health behavior changes," said Rush. Collaborative learning can help with sustainability because collaborative learning helps the community help itself by providing it with tools and resources that meet its particular needs and that reflect the community's culture and concerns.

Villaire commended the roundtable staff for asking the participants before the workshop to identify what they hoped to learn from the workshop, and he hoped the roundtable would continue to do so for future workshops. In his opinion, one lesson from the commissioned review was that there is still work to do to raise awareness in communities about health literacy practices, approaches, programs, and interventions. "Let us continue to build that bridge and help inform people who are working in community-based organizations and doing community-based interventions to start thinking and incorporating health literacy practices and principles," he said. Villaire also highlighted several concepts mentioned during the day, including respecting the communities in which investigators work, listening to the community, understanding that building relationships in the community takes time, and realizing that those developing interventions need to be receptive to change, flexible, and curious. Reflecting on the idea of love, he said that he thinks of putting the needs, requests, and desires of someone else ahead of one's own, and if the field continues to embrace that in its work on health literacy, as well as in life in general, the world would be a better place.

The best people to define community, said Pleasant, are the people who live in it, and the only way to get to a working definition is to go into the community and talk to the people who live there. He also commented on the need to bring together two different paradigms of thought—the medical paradigm and the public paradigm—and getting the medical community and the public to use the same words and have the same goals. The key to accomplishing that is to listen to where people are and use that knowledge to bring people together.

Brach said that she struggles with the evaluation piece of community-based work given that the ultimate goal of evaluation is to find out what does not work, to avoid wasting time and resources, and to spread and scale an intervention that does work. However, as many speakers mentioned throughout the day, interventions need to be tailored to meet the needs of a specific community, raising the question of how applicable the results will be in another community that has its specific needs and characteristics. "That, to me, is something that we have not really tackled today," said Brach.

Elwood said that he believes it is important when speaking to others to describe what community means, given that place or setting do not always equal community. Community, he said, is more about the relationships among people. In his opinion, it is important to describe the composition of a community and account for the relationships among members of the community, how information diffuses through the community, and how the members of the community make decisions. Doing so will improve the health literacy and numeracy processes that go on in that community.

Stacey Rosen from Northwell Health said that although the members of the roundtable come from different places, at the end of the day, every member has the goal of improving the health of the nation's communities and the country as a whole. She said that she loved the emphasis on the words humility and flexibility that she heard throughout the day, and recounted something her dean told the 300 or so senior leaders at Northwell Health's annual diversity meeting. He reminded them not to pat themselves on the back for their community work until the community thanks them, because going into any community and thinking that one knows better is a fast way to fail and lose trust. Rosen also said that rigor in the field is "unbelievably crucial." The health literacy field should look at work from behavioral economics and implementation science to learn about ways of getting communities to adopt effective interventions. "There is a tremendous amount being written now in change management science, which needs to bring rigor into what we do," said Rosen. "We need to bring real science into what works and what does not, and bring our different approaches together."

Logan had two take-home lessons. The first was that the review paper applies as much to health literacy research focused on mental health as it does about community health literacy interventions. His other lesson was that community health literacy intervention research would be improved if evaluation frameworks assessed more of the social and structural determinants of health that affect populations. "It seems to me that progress occurs when we put all of them together," said Logan. "One of the reasons we want to do that is because health literacy is one of the few variables that is both a structural and social determinant of health."

Duhig said that the issues of engaging and motivating members of a community will become easier when every individual has access to all of their health information because that will enable individuals to develop an internal locus of control when it comes to their health. Giving everyone control over their own health information will also start driving longitudinal evaluation studies, he said.

Rosof, offering the final comment on the day, mentioned listening, observing, valuing, and encouraging as important messages, as well as the fact that building sustainably healthy communities and community relationships requires time, respect, love, and flexibility as core competencies. He then adjourned the workshop.

References

Baker, D. W. 2006. The meaning and the measure of health literacy. *Journal of General Internal Medicine* 21(8):878–883.

Chew, L. D., J. M. Griffin, M. R. Partin, S. Noorbaloochi, J. P. Grill, A. Snyder, K. A. Bradley, S. M. Nugent, A. D. Baines, and M. VanRyn. 2008. Validation of screening questions for limited health literacy in a large VA outpatient population. *Journal of General Internal Medicine* 23(5):561–566.

Chibanda, D. 2017. Reducing the treatment gap for mental, neurological and substance use disorders in Africa: Lessons from the friendship bench in Zimbabwe. *Epidemiology and Psychiatric Sciences* 26(4):342–347.

Chibanda, D., T. Bowers, R. Verhey, S. Rusakaniko, M. Abas, H. A. Weiss, and R. Araya. 2015. The friendship bench programme: A cluster randomised controlled trial of a brief psychological intervention for common mental disorders delivered by lay health workers in Zimbabwe. *International Journal of Mental Health Systems* 9:21.

Coleman, C., S. Kurtz-Rossi, J. McKinney, A. Pleasant, I. Rootman, and L. Shohet. 2009. *The Calgary charter on health literacy.* Montreal, Quebec: The Centre for Literacy.

Handley, M. A., E. Harleman, E. Gonzalez-Mendez, N. E. Stotland, P. Althavale, L. Fisher, D. Martinez, J. Ko, I. Sausjord, and C. Rios. 2016. Applying the COM-B model to creation of an IT-enabled health coaching and resource linkage program for low-income Latina moms with recent gestational diabetes: The STAR MAMA program. *Implementation Science* 11(1):73.

Herman, A., and P. Jackson. 2010. Empowering low-income parents with skills to reduce excess pediatric emergency room and clinic visits through a tailored low literacy training intervention. *Journal of Health Communication* 15(8):895–910.

Herman, A., B. B. Nelson, C. Teutsch, and P. J. Chung. 2012. "Eat healthy, stay active!": A coordinated intervention to improve nutrition and physical activity among Head Start parents, staff, and children. *American Journal of Health Promotion* 27(1):e27–e36.

Hernandez, M. Y., and K. C. Organista. 2013. Entertainment-education? A fotonovela? A new strategy to improve depression literacy and help-seeking behaviors in at-risk immigrant Latinas. *American Journal of Community Psychology* 52(3–4):224–235.

IOM (Institute of Medicine). 2004. *Health literacy: A prescription to end confusion.* Washington, DC: The National Academies Press.

IOM. 2011. *Leading health indicators for Healthy People 2020: Letter report.* Washington, DC: The National Academies Press.

Kirkpatrick, D. L. 1959. Techniques for evaluating training programs. *Journal of the American Society of Training Directors* 13(3):21–26.

Kirkpatrick, J. D., and W. K. Kirkpatrick. 2016. *Kirkpatrick's four levels of training evaluation.* Alexandria, VA: ATD Press.

Kuruvilla, S., N. Mays, A. Pleasant, and G. Walt. 2006. Describing the impact of health research: A research impact framework. *BMC Health Services Research* 6:134.

McLeroy, K. R., B. L. Norton, M. C. Kegler, J. N. Burdine, and C. V. Sumaya. 2003. Community-based interventions. *American Journal of Public Health* 93(4):529–533.

Nelson, B. B., C. Teutsch, P. J. Chung, and A. Herman. 2014. Predictors of sustained implementation of low-literacy health education programs. *Journal of Community Medicine and Health Education* 4(314):1–5.

Powers, B. J., J. V. Trinh, and H. B. Bosworth. 2010. Can this patient read and understand written health information? *Journal of the American Medical Association* 304(1):76–84.

Spencer, L. M., M. W. Schooley, L. A. Anderson, C. S. Kochtitzky, A. S. DeGroff, H. M. Devlin, and S. L. Mercer. 2013. Seeking best practices: A conceptual framework for planning and improving evidence-based practices. *Preventing Chronic Disease* 10:E20. http://dx.doi.org/10.5888/pcd10.130186 (accessed February 12, 2018).

Appendix A

Workshop Agenda

Community-Based Health Literacy Interventions: A Workshop
July 19, 2017

8:30–8:45	**Welcome and Workshop Overview** *Bernard Rosof, M.D., Chair, Roundtable on Health Literacy*
8:45–9:15	**Presentation of the Commissioned Paper** *Cynthia Baur, Ph.D.* *Director, Horowitz Center for Health Literacy* *University of Maryland School of Public Health*
9:15–9:45	**Discussion**
9:45–12:15	**Program Presentations with Moderated Discussion to Follow**
9:45–10:05	**Health Literacy in Public Libraries** *Marisa New, M.P.H., OTR* *Board Member, Oklahoma Health Equity Network* *Chair, Southwest Regional Health Equity Council* *Leslie Gelders* *Literacy Coordinator* *Oklahoma Department of Libraries*

10:05–10:20 BREAK

10:20–10:40 **Community-Based Health Literacy Programs**
Catina O'Leary, Ph.D., L.M.S.W.
President and CEO
Health Literacy Media

10:40–11:00 **Health Literacy in Head Start Programs**
Ariella Herman, Ph.D.
Research Director
Johnson & Johnson Health Care Institute
Senior Lecturer, Decisions, Operations, and Technology Management
University of California, Los Angeles, Anderson School of Management

11:00–11:45 **Moderated Panel Discussion with Presenters**
Moderator: *Earnestine Willis, M.D., M.P.H.*
Kellner Professor in Pediatrics
Medical College of Wisconsin

11:45–12:15 **Discussion**

12:15–1:15 LUNCH

1:15–1:20 **Introductions**

1:20–1:40 **Issues and Challenges in Evaluating Community-Based Health Literacy Interventions**
Andrew Pleasant, Ph.D.
Senior Advisor on Health Literacy Interventions, Research, and Evaluation
Health Literacy Media

1:40–2:30 **Moderated Panel Discussion with Evaluators**
Moderator: *Cindy Brach, M.P.P.*
Senior Health Policy Researcher
Agency for Healthcare Research and Quality

Panelists:
Oscar Espinosa, M.A.
Senior Associate
Community Science

Anil Thota, M.P.H.
Associate Director for Systematic Review Science
Systematic Review Team Lead–Community Guide Branch
Centers for Disease Control and Prevention

Sherrie Flynt Wallington, Ph.D.
Assistant Professor of Oncology
Lombardi Comprehensive Cancer Center
Georgetown University Medical Center

2:30–3:00 **Discussion**

3:00–3:15 BREAK

3:15–4:00 **Moderated Dialogue: Where Do We Go from Here?**
Moderator: *Michael Villaire, M.S.L.M.*
CEO, Institute for Healthcare Advancement

Panelists:
Maureen Daniels
Director, Wellness at Work
Berkshire Health Systems

William Elwood, Ph.D.
OppNet Facilitator/Health Scientist Administrator
Office of Behavioral and Social Sciences Research
National Institutes of Health

Michele Erikson
Executive Director
Wisconsin Health Literacy

Caroline Young, M.S.
Executive Director
NashvilleHealth

4:00–4:30	**Roundtable Discussion**
4:30–5:15	**Open Discussion**
5:15–5:45	**Reflections on the Day**
5:45	ADJOURN

Appendix B

Biographical Sketches of Workshop Moderators, Speakers, and Panelists

Cynthia Baur, Ph.D., became the director of the Horowitz Center for Health Literacy at the University of Maryland (UMD) in January 2017. Prior to working at UMD, Dr. Baur worked for 17 years in communication leadership roles with the Centers for Disease Control and Prevention (CDC) in Atlanta and the U.S. Department of Health and Human Services in Washington, DC. Most recently, she served as the senior advisor for health literacy in the CDC Office of the Associate Director for Communication and as CDC's senior official for the Plain Writing Act implementation. During her federal tenure, she led multiple initiatives to define best practices and guidelines in health communication and health literacy. She was the first manager of the Healthy People health communication objectives and the editor of the *U.S. National Action Plan to Improve Health Literacy*. She created CDC's health literacy website, which provides tools and online training to improve health literacy and public health, and she is the co-creator of the CDC Clear Communication Index, a set of scientific criteria for creating clear public communication materials. Her approach is based on communication science and focuses on providing diverse audiences with information in ways that they can understand and use.

Cindy Brach, M.P.P., is a senior health policy researcher at the Agency for Healthcare Research and Quality (AHRQ). She conducts and oversees research on health literacy, cultural and linguistic competence, system design innovations, Medicaid, and the State Children's Health Insurance Program. Ms. Brach spearheads AHRQ's health literacy and cultural competence activities, coordinating AHRQ's work in developing measures, improving the evidence base, and creating implementation tools. She has served on numerous expert panels in these areas for organizations such as the Office of Minority Health, the Joint Commission, the National Quality Forum, and The California Endowment. Ms. Brach also leads the national evaluation of the Children's Health Insurance Program Reauthorization Act Quality Demonstration Grants. Her publications include *New Federal Policy Initiatives to Boost Health Literacy Can Help the Nation Move Beyond the Cycle of Costly "Crisis Care"*; *Evidence on the Chronic Care Model in the New Millennium*; *America's Health Literacy: Why We Need Accessible Health Information*; *Will It Work Here? A Decision Maker's Guide to Adopting Innovations*; and *Integrating Literacy, Culture, and Language to Improve Quality of Health Care for Diverse Populations.* Before working at AHRQ, Ms. Brach was the associate director for research and analysis at the Mental Health Policy Resource Center, where she directed mental health and health policy research projects with an emphasis on managed care. Her earlier health and human services experience includes serving as a welfare reform consultant and provider of technical assistance, a state-level administrator, and a municipal policy analyst. Ms. Brach received her Master of Public Policy degree from the University of California, Berkeley, where she was advanced to Ph.D. candidacy.

Maureen L. Daniels, M.Ed., is the director of wellness at work at Berkshire Health Systems (BHS), where she has designed and implemented programs to improve the health literacy of the community. Berkshire Health Systems is a small community health system nestled in the Berkshire Hills of Massachusetts. It offers wellness programming for its staff and their spouses, community businesses, and the community at large. Ms. Daniels incorporates much of her social service background into the health literacy work in supporting her colleagues. In 2013, BHS partnered with the Canyon Ranch Institute to bring a health literacy curriculum into underserved neighborhoods in Berkshire County. Ms. Daniels oversees the three core teams that have developed since the program's conception. More than 250 community members have already graduated from the program. She earned her bachelor's degree from The State University of New York at Potsdam and her master's degree in Health Promotion and Wellness from Springfield College.

William (Bill) N. Elwood, Ph.D., is the Basic Behavioral and Social Science Opportunity Network (OppNet)/health science administrator in the National Institutes of Health (NIH) Director's Office of Behavioral and Social Sciences Research (OBSSR). OBSSR integrates BSSR within the larger NIH research enterprise and leads research on emerging topics across the agency. For example, OBSSR led a set of health literacy–targeted funding opportunities to ensure that applications in this emerging field received expert, fair, and thorough review. Currently, Dr. Elwood manages NIH's OppNet, a trans-NIH initiative that develops initiatives on basic social-behavioral mechanisms and processes that relate across the disease- and somatic-focused missions of NIH's Institutes and Centers. To date, OppNet has funded 173 unique research projects. Before joining NIH, he was the research and development director for the largest mental health and substance abuse agency in South Florida. During this time, he developed and implemented quality assurance practices that led to the Commission on Accreditation of Rehabilitation Facilities and Medicaid accreditation, supervised the implementation of the Health Insurance Portability and Accountability Act, and collaborated with a local housing authority to provide all clinical and medical supervision services for a family-centered, public housing-based treatment center. Prior to his work in health services, Dr. Elwood held faculty positions at Auburn University and The University of Texas at Houston, where he conducted community-based research throughout the United States and Mexico on substance abuse prevention and treatment, drug use epidemiology, public housing-based health initiatives, sexually transmitted infections/HIV-intervention efficacy studies, and economic self-sufficiency programs. NIH, the Substance Abuse and Mental Health Services Administration, the World Health Organization, the state of Texas, and private foundations supported his research. His publications concentrated on attitudes and beliefs of hard-to-reach populations and the influences that cultural and personal values, as well as community settings, have on mental health, health-related behaviors, risky behaviors, and participation in civic life. His publications in community epidemiology of illegal and diverted substance use remain definitive in clinical, legal, and news fields. Dr. Elwood is the author of 35 peer-reviewed publications and 4 scientific books. He has received multiple NIH Director's awards and two national awards for a research book and article of the year, respectively.

Michele Erikson is the executive director of Wisconsin Literacy, Inc., a coalition providing support and leadership to 75 local literacy agencies. In 2005 she began working in health literacy by directing small community-based projects with local literacy agencies to improve understanding of public health. In 2007 she led the formation of a grassroots regional effort to support health literacy initiatives throughout Wisconsin. In 2010, with three successful statewide health literacy summits completed and additional outside funding, Health Literacy Wisconsin, a division of Wisconsin Literacy, Inc., was launched under her leadership. The work of the division continues on local, regional, and national levels to deliver educational workshops on health information such as influenza, understanding medicines, health insurance, and health access. The division also developed a business plan that provides services to help health care professionals incorporate health literacy strategies into their communication with patients. Wisconsin Literacy continues to host a national Health Literacy Summit every other year.

Oscar J. Espinosa, M.A., is a senior associate at Community Science, a research, evaluation, and development firm in Gaithersburg, Maryland. He is an experienced health services researcher who specializes in the evaluation of programs that deliver services to vulnerable populations, including delivery of language assistance services in public health centers and hospital systems, culturally and linguistically appropriate services in managed care organizations (MCOs), and programs that deliver drug prevention education to recent immigrant families. His career began with extensive field research in the colonies along the U.S.–Mexico border, and he has expanded this work to successfully direct large, multisite evaluation projects for various federal clients, including the U.S. Department of Health and Human Services (HHS), the Corporation for National and Community Service, the Agency for Healthcare Research and Quality, the U.S. Department of Justice, the U.S. Census Bureau, and the U.S. Agency for International Development. For the past 3 years, Mr. Espinosa has directed an evaluation related to the Patient Protection and Affordable Care Act for HHS's Office of Minority Health, which assessed the effectiveness of outreach and education strategies designed to reach and inform underserved populations throughout the country on the benefits of enrolling in health insurance and accessing preventive health services. In addition to his field research, Mr. Espinosa has also completed a national survey to gauge the awareness of racial and ethnic health disparities among the general population and that of practicing physicians, as well as a national survey of MCOs that investigated the nature and extent of culturally and linguistically appropriate services delivered by MCOs.

Leslie A. Gelders is the literacy coordinator at the Oklahoma Department of Libraries (ODL) Literary Resource Office, which is nationally recognized for its support and leadership of statewide literacy efforts. Under the direction of Ms. Gelders, the literacy office works with library- and community-based literacy programs, state agencies, and other organizations to promote literacy throughout Oklahoma. In recent years, ODL has placed a major emphasis on health literacy. With Ms. Gelders's assistance, public libraries and local literacy programs have initiated and enhanced efforts that address Oklahoma's low health ranking. What started as a pilot project of five sites has developed into one of ODL's priorities and is included in the agency's new 5-year plan. Ms. Gelders serves on the steering committee of the Oklahoma Health Equity Campaign, was a two-term president of the Oklahoma Literacy Coalition, and served on a number of state and national literacy committees and governance councils. Her skills in marketing, training, building partnerships, and grant writing have helped strengthen library and community-based programs throughout the state.

Ariella Herman, Ph.D., M.S., is the research director of the Health Care Institute, which is housed at the University of California, Los Angeles (UCLA), Anderson School of Management. Since 2001, she has successfully designed a systematic approach to health promotion intervention in Head Start/preschool community settings. She has developed tools and resources for early childhood programs to lead effective health care training programs through engagement and dissemination of knowledge and to better prepare parents to address the health care needs of their children. She has received numerous recognition and awards, including the Health Literacy Award, "Most Innovative Health Education & Promotion Program" from the Institute of Healthcare Advancement (2009), the Sabra Woolley Memorial Award for Most Highly Rated Abstract, Health Literacy Annual Research Conference (2009), and the Health Literacy Innovation Champions Award from Health Literacy Innovations (2010). Most recently, the UCLA Health Care Institute was named a partner in the Head Start National Center on Early Childhood Health & Wellness. She has been published in various peer-reviewed journals such as *Journal of Community Health*, *Pediatric Emergency Care*, and *Journal of Health Communication*. She has a B.S. in Mathematics from University Paris VII, an M.S. in Engineering from UCLA, and a Ph.D. in Business from the University of Paris IX Dauphine Business School.

S. Marisa New, M.P.H., OTR, is the chair of the Southwest Regional Health Equity Council and a board member of the Oklahoma Health Equity Campaign. Both are community-based partnerships that strive to address health inequities beyond the health community. Ms. New has always been passionate about advocating for persons disadvantaged by conditions that limit their health potential. Ms. New formally began representing her community as a member of the Oklahoma City Mayor's Committee on Disability Concerns. Now, she is an active member of several councils, committees, and coalitions that include the National Association of Chronic Disease Directors Health Equity Council, Oklahoma Governor's Interagency Council on Homelessness, Oklahoma Governor's United We Ride Council, and Oklahoma Alliance for Public Transportation. She is the Oklahoma representative on the American Public Health Association's Governing Council. For several years, she served as the director of the Health Equity & Resource Opportunities Division at the Oklahoma State Department of Health, where she developed partnerships with non-health sectors addressing food security, housing, transportation, and literacy. Today, she is honored to provide occasional supervision to occupational therapy students who are going through the University of Oklahoma's Health Sciences Center Interprofessional Education and Practice Collaborative. Ms. New has an M.P.H. (Health Administration and Policy) from the University of Oklahoma.

Catina O'Leary, Ph.D., M.S.W., serves as the president and CEO of Health Literacy Media (HLM). Under her direction, HLM's service network has expanded to include some of the largest employers in Missouri, including pharmaceutical companies, hospital systems, business coalitions, and community-based organizations. Chosen by the *St. Louis Business Journal* for professional excellence and dedication to the community, Dr. O'Leary is a member of the 2013 class of "40 Under 40" leaders. She was recently selected to join FOCUS St. Louis's 39th Leadership St. Louis class. Before her appointment as CEO of HLM, Dr. O'Leary was a faculty member at the Washington University School of Medicine in the Department of Psychiatry and the Program on Occupational Therapy. At Washington University, her community-engaged research centered on methods to engage underserved populations in health and social service programs. She focused specifically on women's health. Dr. O'Leary is the past president and continues to serve on the board of The Bridge, a drop-in shelter that offers daily meals and basic social services to homeless and at-risk St. Louisans. She also serves as vice president for Magdalene Saint Louis, a nonprofit that helps women who have survived lives of abuse, prostitution, trafficking, and addiction by providing a community where they can recover and rebuild their lives. Dr. O'Leary earned her B.A. in Psychology from the University of Mississippi and M.S.W. and Ph.D. in Social Work from the George Warren Brown School of Social Work at Washington University.

Andrew Pleasant, Ph.D., M.S., is the senior advisor on Health Literacy Interventions, Research, and Evaluation at Health Literacy Media (www.healthliteracy.media). Dr. Pleasant believes that health literacy is one of the most powerful tools to create informed behavior change. Dr. Pleasant has led and participated in hundreds of presentations and trainings in the United States and around the world, primarily on the topics of health literacy and science, risk, and environmental communication. He has taught at Cornell University, Brown University, and Rutgers University. Dr. Pleasant has published numerous peer-reviewed journal articles and technical reports, and is co-author of the book *Advancing Health Literacy: A Framework for Understanding and Action* (2006). Dr. Pleasant holds a B.A. in journalism from Arizona State University, an M.S. in environmental studies from Brown University, and a Ph.D. in communication from Cornell University.

Anil Thota, M.B.B.S., M.P.H., is the lead for the systematic review science team at the Community Guide Branch within the Division for Public Health Information Dissemination at the Centers for Disease Control and Prevention. The Community Guide Branch supports the Community Preventive Services Task Force, an independent panel of public health and prevention experts that issues findings based on systematic reviews of effectiveness and economic evidence of public interventions and policies for decision makers, policy makers, and implementers. Previously at the Community Guide Branch, Dr. Thota led a team of experts focused on prioritizing and evaluating the effectiveness of interventions aiming to reduce morbidity and mortality from cardiovascular disease and conducted a systematic review and meta-analysis of collaborative care to improve delivery of depression care. Dr. Thota has an M.B.B.S. from Manipal University in India and an M.P.H. from the Bloomberg School of Public Health at Johns Hopkins University. Before joining the Community Guide, Dr. Thota worked on evidence-based recommendations and decision making at multiple organizations such as the World Bank, Cochrane South Asia, and Health Quality Ontario.

Michael Villaire, M.S.L.M., is the CEO of the Institute for Healthcare Advancement, a nonprofit health care public charity dedicated to empowering people to achieve better health, with an emphasis on health literacy. Mr. Villaire produces the Institute for Healthcare Advancement's annual Health Literacy Conference. He has written numerous articles and lectures nationally on health literacy. He is the co-author of the textbook *Health Literacy in Primary Care: A Clinician's Guide* and the easy-to-read, self-help health book *What to Do When Your Child Is Heavy*. He is an adjunct faculty member at Brandman University in Irvine, California, where he teaches a health literacy course for the Master of Science in Health Risk and Crisis Communication program. His background includes 20 years as an editor in health care publishing, including peer-reviewed journals in nursing, hospital publications, physician news magazines, and an online health care portal experiment. He has helped redesign and launch several medical and nursing journals, and managed the development of a multimedia, interactive curriculum in critical care. Mr. Villaire earned his bachelor's degree in English and Communications from Western Michigan University, Kalamazoo, Michigan. He earned his M.S. in Science, Organizational Leadership, and Management from the University of La Verne in California. His thesis examined health literacy in community clinics in regard to adequacy of patient education materials.

Sherrie Flynt Wallington, Ph.D., is an assistant professor of oncology and serves as the program director for the Health Disparities Initiative at Georgetown University's Lombardi Cancer Center. Her research interests focus on using community-based participatory research approaches to explore the role of health communication in reducing and eliminating health disparities among minority and underserved populations. Dr. Wallington recently completed a postdoctoral fellowship with the Harvard School of Public Health and the Dana-Farber Cancer Institute. Dr. Wallington attended Howard University and received a Ph.D. in Mass Communication, specializing in Health Communication, and also holds undergraduate and graduate degrees from the University of North Carolina at Greensboro.

Earnestine Willis, M.D., M.P.H., is a Kellner Professor in Pediatrics, director of the Center for the Advancement of Underserved Children, and director of Health Equity and Urban Clinical Care Partnerships. She has nearly three decades of experience in addressing health disparities through the development of successful community initiatives to include research, education, and community services. Her interests include analyzing the impact of systems on children and adolescents, applied public policy, community-oriented programs, medical education, health assessments, and diversity in medicine and child advocacy.

Caroline Young, M.S., is the executive director of NashvilleHealth, an initiative focused on improving the health of the citizens of Nashville-Davidson County. NashvilleHealth is chaired and was created by former U.S. Senate Majority Leader Bill Frist (R-TN) in an effort to address the area's health equity issues and ensure that Nashville continues to be a great place to live and work. Prior to leading NashvilleHealth, Ms. Young served as the president of the Nashville Health Care Council, one of the nation's foremost health care industry associations. Under her leadership, the Council's membership grew to encompass 300 diverse organizations and launched the one-of-a-kind fellows initiative, designed to further the skills of senior business leaders. Prior to joining the Council, she was the founding executive director of Life Science Tennessee (formerly known as the Tennessee Biotechnology Association). She also served as the director of communications and advertising for the State of Tennessee Department of Economic and Community Development. Ms. Young currently serves on the boards of Cumberland Pharmaceuticals and the Center for Non-Profit Management. She is also a member of the Advisory Board of the Washington, DC-based Women Business Leaders of the U.S. Healthcare Industry. Ms. Young holds a B.A. from the University of Mississippi and an M.S. from the University of Tennessee.

Appendix C

A Review and Report of Community-Based Health Literacy Interventions

by

Cynthia Baur, Ph.D.; Lourdes M. Martinez, Ph.D.; Nedelina Tchangalova, M.L.S., AHIP; and Don Rubin, Ph.D.

Commissioned by the Roundtable on Health Literacy
Health and Medicine Division
National Academies of Sciences, Engineering, and Medicine

A REVIEW AND REPORT OF COMMUNITY-BASED HEALTH LITERACY INTERVENTIONS

Cynthia Baur, Ph.D.
Endowed Professor and Director
Herschel S. Horowitz Center for Health Literacy
School of Public Health
University of Maryland, College Park, MD 20742
Phone: (301) 405-0388
Email: cbaur@umd.edu

Lourdes M. Martinez, Ph.D.
Health Communication Specialist
Office of the Associate Director for Communication Science
Centers for Disease Control and Prevention
Atlanta, GA 30345
Email: gmf5@cdc.gov

Nedelina Tchangalova, M.L.S., AHIP
Public Health Librarian
Engineering and Physical Sciences Library
1403 William E. Kirwan Hall
University of Maryland, College Park, MD 20742
Phone: (301) 405-9151
Email: nedelina@umd.edu

Don Rubin, Ph.D.
Emeritus Professor
Department of Communication Studies
University of Georgia
617 Caldwell Hall, Athens, GA 30602
Email: drubin@uga.edu

Corresponding Author: Cynthia Baur, Ph.D.

Disclaimer: The authors are responsible for the content of this article, which does not necessarily represent the views of the National Academies of Sciences, Engineering, and Medicine or the University of Maryland, College Park.

Disclosures: The authors report no significant conflicts or financial disclosures related to this work.

Acknowledgments: Sincere thanks to Dr. Dogan Eroglu and Tom Chapel, M.A., M.B.A., Centers for Disease Control and Prevention, for their guidance on the evaluation framework; Dr. Alice M. Horowitz, University of Maryland, College Park, for guidance on review design and comments on manuscript drafts; three coders who reviewed articles and prepared spreadsheets; and Heather Platter, M.S., University of Maryland, College Park, for help with coding and manuscript review and preparation.

Funding: This work was commissioned by the National Academies of Sciences, Engineering, and Medicine's Health and Medicine Division's Roundtable on Health Literacy.

ABSTRACT

Background: A scoping literature review was conducted to identify and describe the state of the art of community-based health literacy interventions. "Health literacy" and "community" were the core concepts used to identify relevant interventions for review and analysis. "Health literacy," "community," and "community-based" are terms with a range of meanings. The review aimed to find and report those interventions that intentionally brought together groups of people to participate in an intervention that addressed health literacy issues or tried to change health literacy skills, behaviors, status, or other outcomes as defined by researchers.

Methods: Literature searching was conducted using PubMed, selected EBSCO and ProQuest databases, and Web of Science for relevant studies. Gray literature was searched on websites to identify eligible community-based programs. Search results were limited to English publications from June 2010 to 2017, but no limit was applied to geographical location, participants, health topic, or intervention type. Two authors screened titles and abstracts and identified 170 references suitable for full-text analysis. Papers were reviewed using a standard template with descriptive categories about the intervention, and criteria from the Centers for Disease Control and Prevention "Best Practices" for evidence-based practices and *The Guide to Community Preventive Services* study designs.

Results: Of the 2,402 papers located with the search strategy, 74 papers met the inclusion criteria. Of the included papers, 55 reported that intervention communities were selected because of health literacy concerns; 63 reported that health literacy principles or techniques were used for content or program development; 54 used health literacy measures; and 53 included health literacy outcome information. Only two papers reported large-magnitude effects.

Conclusions: A wide range of community-based health literacy interventions provide qualitative and quantitative evidence of positive outcomes; knowledge change was the most common outcome. Interventions can be strengthened in a number of ways to continue to build the body of knowledge about when and how to best address health literacy in community interventions.

Keywords: health literacy, community, community-based interventions

INTRODUCTION

This paper reports the results of a scoping literature review (Arksey and O'Malley 2005) to identify and describe community-based health literacy interventions. The Roundtable on Health Literacy, Health and Medicine Division, National Academies of Sciences, Engineering, and Medicine commissioned the Herschel S. Horowitz Center for Health Literacy, University of Maryland, to review literature published since 2010 and describe the state of the science of community-based health literacy interventions. The roundtable asked for a review that summarized previous work on community-based health literacy interventions; described new interventions; used a published evaluation framework to evaluate interventions; and reported intervention effect sizes, when available. To identify relevant publications, the roundtable also asked the review team to use broad definitions of "community" and "interventions" that could include policy and system levels as well as individual and group-level activities.

The concept and definition of "community" is central to framing this review. As McLeroy and colleagues noted in their editorial on a community-based interventions review paper, "The term *community-based* has a wide range of meanings" (McLeroy et al. 2003, 529). They observe that too often, *community-based* is equivalent to a description of an intervention setting rather than a way to think of communities as relationships and resources for meeting everyday needs. The roundtable referenced the Institute of Medicine (IOM) health literacy report (IOM 2004) and the Agency for Healthcare Research and Quality (AHRQ) updated systematic review (Berkman et al. 2011) as prior reports that included community health literacy interventions. Although neither report defined "community," both used the word to refer to the physical places where people conduct their everyday lives, distinct from hospitals and doctors' offices. Community clinics and care providers seemed to occupy a middle zone between community and clinical care facility. In the IOM report, "community" also referred to social, cultural, and linguistic identity. Both reports included interventions in which the participants acted as individuals, not necessarily with explicit reference to social identities or bonds, and the community component was often a location, such as a community clinic or hospital.

Since these two reports, the Horowitz Center team located one other non-health topic-specific, community-level health literacy intervention review paper. Nutbeam, McGill, and Premkumar (2017, 3) reported that only seven interventions met their criteria to "improve health literacy with community (non-clinical) populations . . . in particular for interventions that are skills-directed and where improved interactive or critical health literacy is targeted as an outcome." Their review uses "population" and "community" as roughly equivalent terms that describe people not engaged with clinical services. Because of differences in inclusion criteria, three (Chervin et al. 2012; Soto Mas, Ji, et al. 2015; Xie 2011) of the seven papers plus one related paper (Fleary 2012) in their review are in the present review.

Given the roundtable's stated interest in a wide-angle review, the lack of a consensus definition for "community-based health literacy intervention," and the Nutbeam team's small number of results, the Horowitz Center team created a broad working definition to help identify studies for this review. The intent was to, at a minimum, identify interventions with an element of "group-ness" either in the researchers' selection of intervention participants or in the intervention itself, such as a voluntary or continuing education class, community activity, or other event that brought people into contact with each other for the health topic or issue. The ideal would have been to find interventions in which groups formed and sustained social identities and bonds as part of the health actions. To be inclusive, the team created the following definition of "community-based health literacy intervention" for the review:

> *Any purposeful, organized activity to help a group of people find, understand, use, or communicate about health information, services, or issues for themselves or their communities.*

The focus on a group component helped the review team distinguish "individual interventions," which were excluded, from "community interventions," which were included. In "individual interventions," individuals were recruited because they met stated demographic characteristics; once they consented, they participated in the intervention as individuals. Examples are one-on-one coaching or counseling; case management; home visits; and individual education to participate in a health screening. If the sole "community" component was that researchers used an organization, such as a community hospital or community health center, to recruit individuals for an individual-based study, the review team excluded the paper. Studies with community health workers (CHWs) often created a "gray zone" when the paper was not clear if the CHWs, a community group, or both were the intended intervention group. Again, to be inclusive, the team included CHW interventions that aimed to improve CHW health literacy either as an endpoint or to intervene in a community. In "community interventions," a group, such as a church congregation, residents of a senior housing complex, or members of a sporting club, shared a location, experience, or interest and participated in at least one group activity during the intervention.

In addition to distinguishing individual from community interventions, the team separated health literacy from health education interventions by looking for an application of the health literacy concept in the selection of the community; measures and outcomes; or material and program design elements. Health literacy is distinct from health education because the former cultivates flexible (and different) skills or processes that people can deploy in response to changing topics and circumstances, and the latter seeks to impart a non-transferable body of information about particular health conditions or practices; however, health education contributes to health literacy.

METHODS

The definition of "community-based health literacy intervention," along with the search terms used in 14 databases (see Tables C-1, C-2, and C-3), yielded 2,402 publications from traditional peer-reviewed academic sources as well as from unconventional sources or the "gray" literature. The team focused on identifying a discernable group of people targeted by the intervention as a primary means to distinguish community from non-community interventions. To be inclusive and provide a broad view of

TABLE C-1 Keywords for Searching the Literature

Concept 1: "Health Literacy"	Concept 2: "Community"	Other Terms for Consideration in Searching the Gray Literature
Main concept	Terms often found in citations: • community based • community dwelling • community level • community sample • community outreach • community based treatment centers • community health worker Locations mentioned in citations: • health fairs • factories • beauty schools • churches • nail salons • bars • family planning clinics • community health centers	Synonyms for "intervention": • intervention • service • program Intended outcomes of the health literacy intervention: • education* • awareness • communication • promotion • knowledge • skills • understanding • comprehension

* In search results, there were variations of "education," such as "adult education," "nutrition education," and "self-management." To be considered for inclusion, citations with all of these terms must cross with health literacy because a large number of publications on chronic disease self-management do not have health literacy aspects.

TABLE C-2 Search Strategies in Commercial Library Databases

	Databases by Vendor	Filters	Queries	Total Results
	EBSCO			
1	Academic Search Complete	Scholarly (peer-reviewed) journals; publication date 2010–2017; English	SU "health literacy" AND (community OR communities) AND AB (education OR awareness OR communication OR promotion OR knowledge OR skills OR understanding OR comprehension) NOT ("information literacy" OR "media literacy" OR "computer literacy" OR "digital literacy")	1,214
2	CINAHL	Academic journals, dissertations, continuing education units Publication date 2010–2017; English	SU "health literacy" AND (community OR communities) AND AB (education OR awareness OR communication OR promotion OR knowledge OR skills OR understanding OR comprehension) NOT ("information literacy" OR "media literacy" OR "computer literacy" OR "digital literacy")	27
3	Education Source	Scholarly (peer-reviewed) journals; publication date 2010–2017; English	SU "health literacy" AND (community OR communities) AND AB (education OR awareness OR communication OR promotion OR knowledge OR skills OR understanding OR comprehension) NOT ("information literacy" OR "media literacy" OR "computer literacy" OR "digital literacy")	373
4	ERIC	Peer reviewed Publication date 2010–2017; English	TI "health literacy" AND (community OR communities) AND AB (education OR awareness OR communication OR promotion OR knowledge OR skills OR understanding OR comprehension) NOT ("information literacy" OR "media literacy" OR "computer literacy" OR "digital literacy")	10

TABLE C-2 Continued

	Databases by Vendor	Filters	Queries	Total Results
5	Health Policy Reference Center	Scholarly (peer-reviewed) journals; publication date 2010–2017; English	SU "health literacy" AND (community OR communities) AND AB (education OR awareness OR communication OR promotion OR knowledge OR skills OR understanding OR comprehension) NOT ("information literacy" OR "media literacy" OR "computer literacy" OR "digital literacy")	486
6	Health Source: Nursing/ Academic Edition	Scholarly (peer-reviewed) journals; publication date 2010–2017; English	SU "health literacy" AND (community OR communities) AND AB (education OR awareness OR communication OR promotion OR knowledge OR skills OR understanding OR comprehension) NOT ("information literacy" OR "media literacy" OR "computer literacy" OR "digital literacy")	633
	EBSCO			
7	Professional Development Collection	Scholarly (peer-reviewed) journals; publication date 2010–2017; English	SU "health literacy" AND (community OR communities) AND AB (education OR awareness OR communication OR promotion OR knowledge OR skills OR understanding OR comprehension) NOT ("information literacy" OR "media literacy" OR "computer literacy" OR "digital literacy")	123
8	PsycINFO	Academic journals, books, dissertations; publication date 2010–2017; English	SU "health literacy" AND (community OR communities) AND AB education OR awareness OR communication OR promotion OR knowledge OR skills OR understanding OR comprehension) NOT ("information literacy" OR "media literacy" OR "computer literacy" OR "digital literacy")	441

continued

TABLE C-2 Continued

	Databases by Vendor	Filters	Queries	Total Results
9	Social Sciences	Scholarly (peer-reviewed) journals; publication date 2010–2017; English	SU "health literacy" AND (community OR communities) AND AB (education OR awareness OR communication OR promotion OR knowledge OR skills OR understanding OR comprehension) NOT ("information literacy" OR "media literacy" OR "computer literacy" OR "digital literacy")	212
10	SocINDEX	Scholarly (peer-reviewed) journals; publication date 2010–2017; English	SU "health literacy" AND (community OR communities) AND AB (education OR awareness OR communication OR promotion OR knowledge OR skills OR understanding OR comprehension) NOT ("information literacy" OR "media literacy" OR "computer literacy" OR "digital literacy")	150
	U.S. National Library of Medicine			
11	PubMed	Publication date 05/01/2010–12/31/2017; English	(((("health literacy"[MeSH Major Topic] OR "health literacy"[Title/Abstract])) AND community) AND ((education[Title/Abstract] OR awareness[Title/Abstract] OR communication[Title/Abstract] OR promotion[Title/Abstract] OR knowledge[Title/Abstract] OR skills[Title/Abstract] OR understanding[Title/Abstract] OR comprehension[Title/Abstract]))) NOT (("information literacy" OR "media literacy" OR "computer literacy" OR "digital literacy"))	752

TABLE C-2 Continued

	Databases by Vendor	Filters	Queries	Total Results
	Thomson Reuters			
12	Web of Science	Timespan: 2010–2017. Indexes: SCI-EXPANDED, SSCI, A&HCI, CPCI-S, CPCI-SSH, BKCI-S, BKCI-SSH, ESCI, CCR-EXPANDED, IC.	TITLE: ("health literacy") AND TITLE: (community OR communities)	76
	ProQuest			
13	Dissertations and Theses Global	Publication date 5/1/10 to 2017; English	SU("health literacy") AND (community OR communities) AND AB(education OR awareness OR communication OR promotion OR knowledge OR skills OR understanding OR comprehension) NOT ("information literacy" OR "media literacy" OR "computer literacy" OR "digital literacy")	142
14	Public Health	Peer reviewed; publication date from 5/1/10 to 2017; English	MeSH("health literacy") AND (community OR communities) AND AB(education OR awareness OR communication OR promotion OR knowledge OR skills OR understanding OR comprehension) NOT ("information literacy" OR "media literacy" OR "computer literacy" OR "digital literacy")	86

TABLE C-3 Detailed Search Strategy in PubMed (performed April 12, 2017)

Search #	Searches	Query	Items Found
#1	Concept 1: "health literacy"	"health literacy"[MeSH Major Topic] OR "health literacy"[Title/Abstract]	4,214
#2	Concept 2: "community"	community	591,711
#3	Intervention outcomes	(education[Title/Abstract] OR awareness[Title/Abstract] OR communication[Title/Abstract] OR promotion[Title/Abstract] OR knowledge[Title/Abstract] OR skills[Title/Abstract] OR understanding[Title/Abstract] OR comprehension[Title/Abstract]	1,733,538
#4	Key terms excluded from results	"information literacy" OR "media literacy" OR "computer literacy" OR "digital literacy"	2,338
#5	(1 AND 2 AND 3) NOT 4	(((("health literacy"[MeSH Major Topic] OR "health literacy"[Title/Abstract])) AND community) AND ((education[Title/Abstract] OR awareness[Title/Abstract] OR communication[Title/Abstract] OR promotion[Title/Abstract] OR knowledge[Title/Abstract] OR skills[Title/Abstract] OR understanding[Title/Abstract] OR comprehension[Title/Abstract]))) NOT (("information literacy" OR "media literacy" OR "computer literacy" OR "digital literacy"))	742

the science, the team allowed "health literacy" to describe the community, intervention, or measures and outcomes.

The following definitions guided the search strategy:

- **Community-based health literacy intervention:** Any purposeful, organized activity to help a group of people find, understand, use, or communicate about health information, services, or issues for themselves or their communities.
- **Health literacy:** Both how people find, process, understand, and communicate about health information and services to protect and promote their health, *and* how organizations and systems support or hinder people in these activities (modified definition from Healthy People, U.S. National Library of Medicine, and *National*

Action Plan to Improve Health Literacy) (*Healthy People 2020* n.d.; HHS 2010; Selden et al. 2000).

The aim for the scoping review was to identify community-based health literacy interventions that have been developed, implemented, and evaluated after the Institute of Medicine health literacy report (IOM 2004) and the evidence review from AHRQ (Berkman et al. 2011). A literature search was conducted based on the guidelines outlined in Arksey and O'Malley's scoping review framework (2005) and the PRISMA flow diagram for reporting standards in systematic reviews and meta-analyses (Moher et al. 2009). Three sets of conceptual key terms were developed in various combinations and Boolean operators to search electronic databases for peer-reviewed publications and gray literature (see Table C-1). The librarian (Tchangalova) designed different search strategies in close cooperation with the first two authors (Baur, Martinez) (see Table C-2). The initial search was conducted using PubMed, 10 EBSCO databases, 2 Proquest databases, and Thomson Reuters' Web of Science. These databases were selected because they offer extensive indexing of relevant literature, such as conference proceedings, reports, theses, and dissertations. After reaching unanimous consensus on the search strategies, the librarian ran the searches on April 21, 2017.

The inclusion and exclusion criteria for the initial search and subse-

TABLE C-4 Criteria for the Inclusion and Exclusion of Papers in the Review

Inclusion	Exclusion
1. Published in English	1. Conceptual models
2. Published between June 2010 and May 2017	2. Associations between health literacy and another concept or variable
3. Peer-reviewed articles (exceptions are theses, dissertations, web pages, posters, and professional/trade publications when enough information was included)	3. Intervention development or protocols
	4. Formative research
	5. Interventions focused on health care professionals or individuals (not groups)
4. Used a community sample	6. Questionnaire or other instrument development
5. "Health literacy" and "community" common terms	7. "Health literacy" and "community" absent in abstract
	8. Health knowledge or skills without a health literacy connection
	9. Community locations or settings, such as health center, used only for recruitment
	10. Review articles, but reference lists were searched for articles meeting inclusion criteria

quent refinements to the sample are in Table C-4. In commercial library databases, searches were limited to peer-reviewed studies published in English during the time frame of June 2010–May 2017. This time span was chosen to identify any new programs developed after the two reports by IOM (2004) and Berkman et al. (2011). Common terms across all databases included "health literacy" and "community." The key term "health literacy" was available in the controlled vocabulary in the majority of the databases, and the search was limited to that particular field. In all other instances, "health literacy" was limited to title or abstract fields.

Gray literature was searched using databases such as MedNar, EthOS, OpenDOAR, and Worldwidescience. The search terms included a combination of key terms as presented in Table C-1. Additional references were obtained by exploring the links listed on the PHPartners web site (PHPartners 2017), as well as library catalogs. In addition, all references of relevant review articles identified in the initial database searches were screened to find additional studies for inclusion.

Process to Select Papers and Conduct Full-Text Review

All references from the initial search were imported in Zotero, a citation management software, and duplicates were removed. References from Zotero were exported to Rayyan, a screening software for systematic reviews, which was used for screening titles and abstracts (Ouzzani et al. 2016). Rayyan caught duplicates that were not initially flagged by Zotero, and the librarian resolved these. The first two authors independently screened the titles and abstracts in Rayyan. They jointly reviewed and discussed 33 percent of the references identified for inclusion and reached consensus. Next, they independently double-reviewed the remaining references and reached consensus by discussion for inclusion. Entries without abstracts were included in the pool of references if the title seemed to fit the inclusion criteria. During the title and abstract review, the first two authors identified eight abstracts containing only protocols, descriptions of future projects, or projected results. The public health librarian followed up with authors to obtain related publications. Only one author had published results, but the study was not included in the final results. The first two authors also identified twenty review articles; the librarian reviewed the reference lists and added studies that met the inclusion criteria.

After the title and abstract screening, the first two authors trained three coders to use a template to review and record information from the full-text articles (see Tables C-5, C-6, and C-7). The template included criteria from the roundtable's initial call for a review paper, the Centers for Disease Control and Prevention's (CDC's) "Seeking Best Practices: A Conceptual Framework for Planning and Improving Evidence-Based Practices" (Spencer

TABLE C-5 Codes and Directions for Community-Based Health Literacy Intervention Review

Intervention Basics		
Background Questions	Coding Label	Coding Directions
What is the intervention?	Description	Record a one- or two-sentence description of the intervention. Record the type of intervention: individual-level; group-level; community-level; system-level; or policy-level. People recruited from communities to participate in educational sessions or classes should be coded as group-level.
What is the topic?	Topic	Record the intervention's topic, such as dementia, HIV, or mental health.
What is the health literacy definition used?	Definition	Record the author's health literacy definition, including all variations using "literacy"; if none is provided, record "none."
What are the format, delivery method, and setting?	Format	Record the format, including number of times intended target population was exposed, duration of exposure, and total length of time intervention was in the field; delivery method, such as counseling, group presentations, community meetings, class, or mass media; and setting, such as community center, place of worship, clinic, or neighborhood; examples are not exhaustive and record all available descriptive details.
Did the intervention team use health literacy instruments?	Instruments	Record yes or no and list the instrument(s) used to measure health literacy, including all variations using "literacy."
When and where did the intervention happen?	Time and place	Record the year(s) when the intervention happened and any location details, such as city, state, or country names; if none provided, record "none."

NOTES: All coding is about the intervention and its results, not an evaluation of the intervention (e.g., for the "description" coding label, describe the intervention, not the evaluation of the intervention; record the intervention reach, not the evaluation reach). "Author statement" means the information is explicitly written in the paper.

TABLE C-6 Centers for Disease Control and Prevention Best Practices Framework

Public Health Impact Elements/ Questions	Coding Label	Coding Directions
Effectiveness: Extent to Which the Intervention Achieves the Desired Outcomes		
What are the intervention's desired outcomes?	Desired outcomes	Record and label intended primary and other outcomes provided by authors; if none are provided and the paper is exploratory or a needs assessment, remove paper from pool.
To what extent does the intervention achieve the desired outcomes?	Achieved outcomes	Record and label achieved primary and other outcomes provided by authors.
What is the magnitude of the effect?	Magnitude	For quantitative outcomes, record the magnitude of effect and confidence intervals by primary and other outcomes; if no quantitative results, record "none."
What is the outcome's significance to public health, systems, or organizational outcomes?	Significance	Record any author statements about how important the intervention's outcome is for public health, systems, or organizational outcomes; if no author statements, record "none."
What are the intervention's benefits or risks?	Benefits/risks	Record any author statements about how the intended target population benefited from the intervention or was put at risk or harmed by the intervention; if no author statements, record "none."
Does the intervention promote health equity?	Health equity	Record any author statements about how the intervention affected health disparities or health equity; if no author statements, record "none."

TABLE C-6 Continued

Public Health Impact Elements/ Questions	Coding Label	Coding Directions
Reach: Extent to Which the Intervention Affects Intended and Critical Target Population(s)		
What is the intervention's intended and critical target population?	Intended population	Record all details of the intended and critical target population. Details may include, but are not limited to, gender, age, race/ethnicity, socioeconomic status, preferred language, and literacy skill level. Record if the intervention targeted individuals with similar issues, concerns, or information or service use, such as a community clinic; groups, such as families or community members in a class; or general community members defined by location, cultural identity, or other group characteristic.
To what extent does the intervention reach the intended and critical target population?	Reach	Record all information about people and communities recruited for and completing the intervention, including control groups; if provided, report proportion of the intended population actually reached and potential reach of the intervention.
How representative are the people or communities reached through the intervention compared with those ultimately affected by the problem?	Representativeness	Record any author statements, positive or negative, about population representativeness; information may be located in limitations discussion; if no author statements, record "none."
Feasibility: Extent to Which the Intervention Can Be Implemented		
What are the barriers to implementation?	Barriers	Record any author statements about barriers to implementing the intervention; if no author statements, record "none."
What are the facilitators to implementation?	Facilitators	Record any author statements about facilitators or what made it easier to implement the intervention; if no author statements, record "none."
Which resources are necessary to fully implement the intervention?	Resources	Record any author statements about resources, such as facilities, personnel, or materials, to implement the intervention; if no author statements, record "none."
What is the cost-effectiveness of the intervention?	Cost-effectiveness	Record any author statements about costs or cost-effectiveness of the intervention; if no author statements, record "none."

continued

TABLE C-6 Continued

Public Health Impact Elements/ Questions	Coding Label	Coding Directions
Sustainability: Extent to Which the Intervention Can Be Maintained and Achieve Desired Outcomes Over Time		
	Sustainability	Record any author statements about how the intervention did or could continue past the initial implementation; if no author statements, record "none."
Transferability: Extent to Which the Intervention Can Be Applied to or Adapted for Various Contexts		
	Transferability	Record any author statements about other contexts in which the intervention was tried or adapted for use; include details of adaptations if provided; if no author statements, record "none."

TABLE C-7 Drop-Down Lists for the Cells

Study Design	Coding Label	Notes
Randomized trial (experiment)	Randomized trial	
Non-randomized "trial" with one or more comparison groups	Non-random trial	
Cohort study	Cohort	
Case-control study	Case-control	
Time series study	Time	
Before–after study	Before–after	Include pre- and posttest questionnaires here
Cross-sectional study	Cross	
Non-comparative study	Non-compare	
Other	Other	

et al. 2013), and the *Guide to Community Preventive Services* study design categories (HHS 2001). Based on the full-text information, both the coders and the first two authors excluded additional articles because they did not include anything about health literacy, a community, and an intervention in the body of the paper. Once coding was complete, the first two authors reviewed and synthesized information on the remaining studies.

RESULTS

The literature search yielded 2,402 non-duplicate records for "health literacy" and "community" (see Figure C-1). Title and abstract review reduced the number to 170 articles for full-text review. The full-text review reduced the final corpus to 74 articles that met the inclusion criteria (see Table C-4 for the criteria and Table C-8 for the 74 articles). Of the included papers, 55 reported that the intervention communities were selected because of health literacy concerns; 63 reported that health literacy principles or techniques were used for content or program development; 54 used health literacy measures; and 53 included health literacy outcome information (Note: one paper could include one to four of the health literacy elements).

A majority (63 percent) of excluded results at the title and abstract stage included "knowledge" in the title or abstract; 16 percent included "skill." Some abstracts mentioned health literacy, but the papers themselves did not treat health literacy in a substantive way; those papers were excluded. Other papers included health literacy only in the background discussion about the need for interventions; others concluded that health literacy had affected their results. In neither case did the authors explicitly address health literacy in the main intervention discussion, and the papers were excluded.

Mental health was the most frequent topic of the final set of papers. The review team chose to include the mental health literacy papers for two reasons. First, the interventions not only intended to develop community members' knowledge of mental health symptoms and conditions, but also their skills to communicate and support others experiencing a mental health condition. Second, the review yielded a significant number of articles on mental health literacy, and the number of articles and variety of groups involved are important findings in themselves. Nutbeam and colleagues (2017, 4) excluded mental health literacy articles in their review because of "significant inconsistencies in the definition of mental health literacy and wide variation in measurement instruments." Definitional inconsistencies are not specific to mental health papers, however, and readers will find variability in how health literacy is defined. Additionally, studies focused on health literacy varied in the use of established, standardized instruments or researcher-created instruments. For these reasons, the papers on mental health literacy did not seem noticeably different from other papers in the review.

The results were clustered by approaches to health literacy improvement, settings, and health topics. The one policy intervention is reported separately. The team chose not to report by community to avoid stigmatization that might come from calling out specific groups as having "low

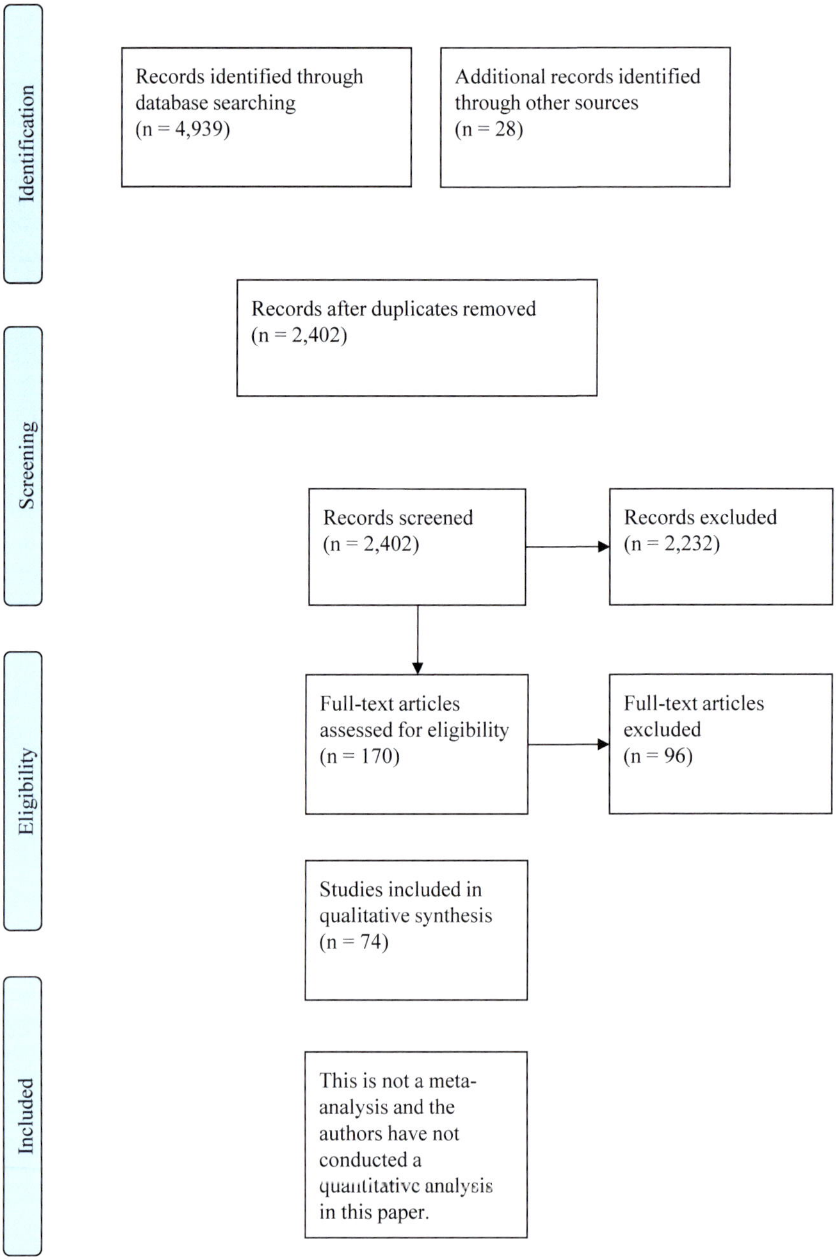

FIGURE C-1 Flowchart for selection of papers for full-text review.

health literacy." Moreover, the lack of significant details about many of the intervention groups made it difficult to create meaningful community categories. As a convenience for readers, Table C-9 reports the frequency of common labels researchers used to describe their intervention communities. Some papers may be counted in more than one category, and not all communities may be represented in the table.

Magnitude of Intervention Effects

The roundtable asked the review team to report the magnitude of intervention effects when available. To assess magnitude, the team relied on reported effect sizes for statistically significant comparisons. One consequence of this methodological decision is that the results table (Table C-8) does not include information on the amount of impact suggested by qualitative analyses. Notwithstanding that decision, the team acknowledges the value of those qualitative analyses, especially when trying to reflect with fidelity the perspectives and experiences of community members. The results table adopts the convention of characterizing effect sizes as small, medium, large, or very large. These characterizations are based on conventional standards for Cohen's d effect sizes, for standardized regression weights (Cohen 1988; Sawilowsky 2009), and for odds ratios (Chen, Cohen, and Chen 2010). Of studies with quantitative outcomes that might have reported effect sizes, 84 percent (59) did not do so. Transparency about magnitude of effects is necessary for rational allocation of public health resources. The failure to calculate and disclose magnitude of effects is contrary to guidelines for reporting experiments (e.g., APA 2010).

Effect sizes that were reported were mainly small, or small to moderate, varying by outcome measure. Only two studies reported any effects that attained a large magnitude. One used fotonovelas with Latinas at a high risk of depression and found large effects of the intervention on knowledge of depression and efficacy to seek help for that condition (Hernandez and Organista 2013). Another achieved very large magnitude increases in breast cancer and cervical cancer screening among Korean Americans by conducting a single educational session led by community health workers (Han et al. 2017).

Health Literacy Skill and Capacity Building

Seven articles reported interventions to improve or increase a group's health literacy skills or an organization's capacity to serve its clients or constituents; an eighth related paper on Ethiopian immigrants in Israel is

(text continues on page 190)

TABLE C-8 Included Studies

Author	Community	Setting	Topic	Intervention
Anderson and Pierce 2012	Intervention focused on coaches and leaders of sports teams as a means of reaching particularly young males in rural communities who might otherwise not be reached by a mental health literacy (MHL) initiative	Football/netball coach training in rural Victoria, Australia	Mental health	Community MHL program focused on sports team coaches and other club leaders to assist them in providing Mental Health First Aid (MHFA) by improving their understanding of mental health conditions, increasing their confidence to assist those with mental illness and decrease stigmatizing attitudes. Two phases from 2007–2009. Training length not discussed.

Health Literacy Component	Study Design	Outcomes	Magnitude
Measures Content Outcomes	Before–after study	At pretraining, 51% felt "not at all confident" or "a little bit confident" to help someone experiencing mental illness. Following training, 90% felt "moderately confident" or "quite a bit confident" that they could help ($p < 0.0010$). Numbers of who correctly identified depression and schizophrenia/psychosis vignettes: depression 73% pretraining, 92% posttraining ($p = 0.007$). psychosis 35% pretraining, 77% posttraining ($p = 0.003$).	Not reported

continued

TABLE C-8 Continued

Author	Community	Setting	Topic	Intervention
Armstrong et al. 2011	Rural community health workers with little understanding of mental health, participants were 21 to 59 years old, majority female, and married, half the participants (46.9%) had not completed high school	Rural Bangalore district, India	Mental health	Mental health training program intended to serve as introductory education to community health workers. Intervention included in-person training and a manual covering introduction to mental health and disorders, mental health first aid, practice-based skills, and mental health promotion. Training in three groups of 23–24 participants by two facilitators between May and October 2010. Training is a four-day course. Adapted MHL survey.

Health Literacy Component	Study Design	Outcomes	Magnitude
Measures Content Outcomes	Before–after study	Percentage of participants able to correctly identify depression and psychosis increased from 22.7% preintervention to 43.9% 3 months following intervention ($p \leq 0.05$). Percentage of participants using potentially useless pharmacologics, such as vitamins including tonics and herbal medicines, appetite stimulants, and sleeping pills decreased 3 months following intervention ($p < 0.001$).	Not reported

continued

TABLE C-8 Continued

Author	Community	Setting	Topic	Intervention
Ayub et al. 2015	Lower health literacy (HL), education, and socioeconomic status (SES) women in Pakistan, ages 15 to 46 years	Vocational training site provided by local nongovernmental organization (NGO)	Civic responsibility, communication skills, iron-deficiency anemia (IDA)	A service learning intervention designed to increase HL about IDA among college students as well as community members. 30-item questionnaire developed to assess HL. Training was an 8-hour session led by 13 trained students in small groups of 5-6 participants.
Beauchamp et al. 2017	See article for details	9 rural/metropolitan, small/large hospitals, community health centers, or municipalities	HL, Ophelia approach	Ophelia Victoria used a participatory design process. Each of nine sites identified different needs and approaches to improving HL in their community. Interventions included reforming health care navigation systems, training for web-based health information searching, and direct instruction in HL. Used Health Literacy Questionnaire (HLQ).

Health Literacy Component	Study Design	Outcomes	Magnitude
Community Measures Content Outcomes	Before–after study	Knowledge about causes and symptoms of IDA and about sources of iron increased following the intervention, particularly among women who had completed at least high school.	Not reported
Measures Content Outcomes	Before–after study	Outcomes varied across sites and intervention approaches, but included increases in selected HL scores.	For 6 sites that reported pretest-to-posttest changes in HLQ scores, effect sizes varied from zero for subscales 4, 5, and 9 to small for subscales 2 and 8, to moderate for subscales 2, 5, 6, and 7.

continued

TABLE C-8 Continued

Author	Community	Setting	Topic	Intervention
Bertera 2014	Community-dwelling African Americans, older adults, lower HL	Local community setting for group education	Diabetes and cardiovascular disease (CVD)	Educational intervention using storytelling slideshows with images/narration from community members to increase awareness of diabetes prevention and management, high blood pressure (HBP), and CVD among older, lower SES African Americans. Three-year study. Intervention was administered in educational sessions lasting 2.5 to 3 hours. Low HL tested using 16-item instrument.
Brown, Collie-Akers, and Fernandez-Ortega 2015	Limited resource, low-literacy Mexican English-language learners, specifically women	Supplemental Nutrition Assistance Program (SNAP) conducted by community health workers (CHWs)	Nutrition literacy	Train-the-trainer model, using CHWs and existing SNAP-Ed nutrition curriculum to help Mexican-immigrant, English-learner women to improve nutrition literacy.

Health Literacy Component	Study Design	Outcomes	Magnitude
Community Measures Content Outcomes	Non-randomized trial	Eating decision scores, knowledge of HBP, and self-efficacy (SE) in those two domains increased from pre- to posttest ($p < 0.001$) for the intervention group. Greatest benefit for lowest HL and oldest participants ($p < 0.01$).	Not reported
Community Content	Before–after study	At the end of the series, participants lost 35 cumulative pounds. All expressed their intention to share their newly learned nutrition literacy skills.	Not reported

continued

TABLE C-8 Continued

Author	Community	Setting	Topic	Intervention
Burgette 2016	Early Head Start (EHS) parents and children under 3 years old	EHS program	Oral health	EHS teachers and staff trained to promote better oral health outcomes among children and families. Curriculum focused on oral health during pregnancy, baby teeth, steps for a healthy smile, classroom tooth-brushing program, and oral health preventive services.
Burghardt et al. 2013	Urban, minority, economically disadvantaged population, primarily African American	Community pharmacy	Medicine literacy and communication skills	Interactive educational board games played in a health party setting. The health party included educational games, health screening booths, music, and prizes. Event done to encourage community members to ask their pharmacists for medication advice. Event was in two major aisles of pharmacy for 4 hours.

Health Literacy Component	Study Design	Outcomes	Magnitude
Community Content	Non-randomized trial	EHS children were more likely to have a dental visit and less likely to have negative quality-of-life effects than children in the Medicaid control group. Results showed similar improvements in dental use regardless of parents' HL levels.	Moderating effect of HL was nil.
Community Content	Before–after study	Game participants were significantly more likely than the control group to indicate they would seek pharmacist medication advice in the future ($p = 0.03$), potential for drug–drug interactions ($p < 0.001$), aware of coupons ($p = 0.01$), and pharmacist review ($p = 0.01$).	Not reported

continued

TABLE C-8 Continued

Author	Community	Setting	Topic	Intervention
Castañeda et al. 2016	Mexican heritage, Spanish-speaking, Latina women (over 40) living in the southern border region of San Diego	Community health center	HL, breast cancer	Health education program delivered via a culturally tailored Spanish cooking class series, Nuestra Codina: Mesa Buena, Vida Sana delivered by a CHW. Sessions were on (1) women's health and cancer basics, (2) HL and navigation of screening services, (3) dispelling breast cancer (BC) myths, (4) communicating with providers, (5) risk reduction strategies, and (6) graduation. Used Chew Health Literacy Screener and Newest Vital Sign (NVS) Assessment Tool.
Chan 2012[a]	Older adults with one or more chronic diseases in Hong Kong	Community centers	Chronic disease	Chronic disease self-management program is delivered in six 2.5-hour group sessions by a professional or lay person.

Health Literacy Component	Study Design	Outcomes	Magnitude
Community Measures Content Outcomes	Before–after study	Participants increased cancer knowledge, nutrition-related behavior/skills, self-reported cancer screenings from pre- to posttest. BC knowledge increased; participants more likely to have cancer screening at posttest and correctly read a nutrition label. No change in BC cultural beliefs, HL, and screening intentions.	Not reported
Community Content	Non-randomized trial	After adjusting for demographic variables, the intervention group had significant improvements in all self-management behaviors and SE outcomes, and 5 of 10 health status measures (all $p < 0.05$). The health care use was not affected by the intervention. Older lay leaders and professionally trained leaders were equally effective.	Illiteracy/low education level interacted with the treatment on fatigue level such that low-literacy individuals who received the intervention obtained a disproportionately high level of fatigue reduction. The effect size for this interaction was moderate.

continued

TABLE C-8 Continued

Author	Community	Setting	Topic	Intervention
Chan 2012[a]	Older adults with non-insulin–dependent diabetes in Hong Kong	Community centers	Diabetes	Diabetes mellitus self-management program had eight weekly 2-hour sessions that delivered disease-related information, teaching and practicing routine self-management tasks and generic self-management skills, enhancing psychosocial support, promoting exercise, and modifying unrealistic beliefs and negative attitudes toward disease.
Chang et al. 2015	Primary and middle school students in Taiwan and their teachers	Schools	Medicine literacy	Community pharmacist and school partnership program to enhance teachers' capacities in implementing correct medication use education. Goal was to enhance teacher and student competencies. Self-administered online questionnaire developed on five core abilities for correct medication use and pain medication literacy.

Health Literacy Component	Study Design	Outcomes	Magnitude
Community Content	Randomized trial	The intervention group improved in diabetes knowledge more than the control group ($p < 0.0005$). Significant reductions of total caloric ($p = 0.018$) and saturated fat intakes ($p = 0.03$) were also found for the intervention group only.	Not reported
Content Measures Outcomes	Non-randomized trial	Program in primary and middle schools significantly enhanced students' knowledge, SE, and skills in correct medication use and pain medication literacy ($p < 0.001$).	Not reported

continued

TABLE C-8 Continued

Author	Community	Setting	Topic	Intervention
Chervin et al. 2012	Adult learners, primarily of color, and immigrant and low-income populations	Six adult education centers	Adult learners' HL skills	HL instruction in adult education curricula to increase adult learners' HL; capacity building of adult education centers' teaching of HL skills. Used Spanish-Test of Functional Health Literacy in Adults (TOFHLA).
Creech 2014	Older adults dwelling in an independent living facility	Retirement community	Medication management	Brief low-HL tailored single intervention, established within monthly health education seminar series, on medication management issues. Content was anecdotal/game show formats. Used NVS.
David et al. 2017	Community members in Tulsa	Churches, YMCA	Antibiotic use/ resistance	Thirty-minute education sessions addressed appropriate antibiotic use and how to reduce resistance. Used NVS.

Health Literacy Component	Study Design	Outcomes	Magnitude
Community Measures Content Outcomes	Before–after study	HL scores increased from pretest to posttest for both English as a second language (ESL) and non-ESL adult basic education students ($p < 0.001$). Qualitative analyses suggested that the intervention also enhanced SE.	Not reported
Community Measures Content Outcomes	Before–after study	The intervention more than doubled knowledge scores in 100% of participants. However, SE scores were not significantly changed.	Not reported
Measures Content Outcomes	Before–after study	Average score on antibiotic knowledge test increased following the intervention ($p < 0.005$).	Not reported

continued

TABLE C-8 Continued

Author	Community	Setting	Topic	Intervention
Diamond et al. 2011	Low-income, minority youth from third to eighth grade (pilot study focused on urban communities of high need: at risk for chronic disease and qualified for no-cost lunches)	After-school program	Chronic disease and substance abuse	Building Wellness is a youth HL 6-year curriculum targeting low-income youth from third to eighth grade. Lessons on asthma, obesity/overweight, accidental injury, and drug/alcohol use. REALM-Teen assessment tool used.
Dowrick et al. 2013	Older immigrants, especially from Somalia, Pakistan, and Bangladesh	Varied across seven sites, including a community center	Mental health	The AMP Development Partnership was a multifaceted model incorporating local communities, primary care teams, and well-being therapists. The final element of the project was a psychosocial intervention with three arms: individual intervention, group intervention, and "signposting" to available services.

Health Literacy Component	Study Design	Outcomes	Magnitude
Community Content Measures Outcomes	Before–after study	Program increased knowledge and retention of information across years. Instructor reports show positive behavior change and an increase in curiosity about health and the body. Participants reported regularly checking nutrition labels of their snacks, washing their hands without prompting, and asking their doctor questions during appointments. Based on observations, participants display SE and confidence in their ability to deal with health issues.	Not reported
Content	Randomized trial	The intervention revealed no statistically significant differences relative to usual care for the measured outcomes: self-reported well-being, depression, anxiety, functioning, and overall health. Qualitative findings were encouraging.	Not reported

continued

TABLE C-8 Continued

Author	Community	Setting	Topic	Intervention
Fleary 2012	Mothers of young children in Head Start, EHS programs	Familiar community locations	Caretakers' HL and child wellness with respect to diet and nutrition, physical activity, and sleep	A module-based intervention focusing on helping mothers with children in Head Start programs to understand what it means to eat right, get sufficient physical activity and sleep, engage in healthy parenting, and manage stress and mental wellness for themselves and their children. Intervention materials were informed by members of the community and Head Start programs. Developed own measure for HL. Study completed in three phases over a 2-year period. Four group interventions, intervention was five sessions, 1.5 hours each.
Flecha, García, and Rudd 2011	Children and parents in low-SES, immigrant, and cultural minority areas connected to local schools	Preprimary and primary schools in Spain	HL skills	Health programs with different topics for school children at six schools and parents in the surrounding community.

Health Literacy Component	Study Design	Outcomes	Magnitude
Community Measures Content Outcomes	Before–after study	Knowledge of the relationship between nutrition and disease and parental encouragement of child physical activity declined following the intervention ($p < 0.05$). General knowledge and beliefs about nutrition, about physical activity, and about sleep hygiene at posttest and at delayed posttest exceeded pretest ($p < 0.05$). Reported increases in children's vegetable and fruit intake increased from pretest to posttest ($p < 0.05$). Knowledge about relationship between stress and physical health increased from pretest to posttest ($p < 0.05$).	For all significant pretest to posttest changes, effect sizes were small.
Community Measures Outcomes	Case study	Qualitative analysis suggested that community-based approaches helped vulnerable families make health decisions and gain access to and use health care services.	Not applicable

continued

TABLE C-8 Continued

Author	Community	Setting	Topic	Intervention
Freedman 2011	Adult African American learners in an adult education class	Adult literacy center in Atlanta, Georgia	HL skills	Classes over a 12-week period with two classes per week, each 2 hours long, to teach functional HL skills to adult learners.
Fung et al. 2016	Hong Kong Chinese adolescent students and adults	School and community-based service	Mental health	Five 3.5-hour workshops facilitated by volunteers. The program also provided direct contact/service opportunities with people recovering from mental illness and required design of school-based mental health promotion materials. Self-developed measures.

Health Literacy Component	Study Design	Outcomes	Magnitude
Community Measures Outcomes	Case study	Multiple strategies from cognitive psychology and adult learning theories help adults learn HL skills and carry health behavior change into everyday life.	Not applicable
Content Measures Outcomes	Other: posttest only with comparison group	At posttest student and adult/volunteer participants had a higher level of MHL and lower level of stigma toward individuals with mental illness, compared with those who did not participate in the program.	Not reported

continued

TABLE C-8 Continued

Author	Community	Setting	Topic	Intervention
Goeman et al. 2016	Older adults with diabetes in community housing receiving home nursing support	Nursing homes	Diabetes, HL	Ophelia approach supports health care services and providers to co-design interventions that are responsive to the HL needs of their client. The project encompasses nine diverse health care services, but this study focuses on a home nursing service. This intervention included materials and training for home nursing service nurses and client materials for diabetes education and support. Used HLQ.

Health Literacy Component	Study Design	Outcomes	Magnitude
Community Measures Content Outcomes	Before–after study	Diabetes Knowledge Questionnaire scores did not change due to the intervention. Scores on two HLQ subscales—sufficient information to manage health and understanding health information sufficiently to guide action—did increase from pre- to posttest.	Small effect sizes were found for increments in the two HLQ subscales that showed increases following the intervention. As predicted, zero effect was found on subscale 5 (appraisal of health information).

continued

TABLE C-8 Continued

Author	Community	Setting	Topic	Intervention
Goodman, Dias, and Stafford 2010	Community leaders, including community health workers, leaders of faith- and community-based organizations, and community members improving minority health	Libraries in Suffolk County, New York	Scientific and research literacy	Community Alliance for Research Empowering Social Change (CARES) training was an academic and community partnership consisting of a 15-week public health curriculum to train community members about evidence-based public health, increase community members' scientific literacy, and develop the infrastructure for community-based participatory research to analyze and address health disparities in the community. Included 11 didactic 3-hour training sessions and 4 experiential workshops.

Health Literacy Component	Study Design	Outcomes	Magnitude
Content	Before–after study	Posttest showed CARES Fellows increased their knowledge and understanding of research ($p < 0.005$). Qualitative analysis showed that participants increased their capacity to participate as research partners. Ten of the thirteen Fellows submitted pilot grant proposals for feedback.	Not reported

continued

TABLE C-8 Continued

Author	Community	Setting	Topic	Intervention
Gray, Elliott, and Wale 2013	Adults (18+) responding to ad for free community workshops to improve ability to find/use online health information	Public library in major Australian city	Health information–seeking skills	A team of clinicians, consumer representatives, and librarians provided 11 2-hour workshops for adults to improve their ability to find and use evidence-based health information online.
Han et al. 2017	Adult (18+) Korean American women attending 1 of 23 ethnic churches in Washington, DC, Maryland, and Baltimore metro areas	Church	Mammogram, Pap smear	This study was designed to test a community health worker intervention to increase mammogram and Pap screening among Korean American women. CHWs delivered HL skills training in 1.5- to 2-hour meeting. Used Assessment of Health Literacy in Cancer Screening.

Health Literacy Component	Study Design	Outcomes	Magnitude
Content	Before–after study	97% of participants agreed/ strongly agreed the workshop improved knowledge of and skills to find and use evidence-based health information; 78% strongly agreed/agreed the workshop improved their attitude toward information; and 93% strongly agreed/agreed the workshop would change the way they access health information online. After the workshops, people also said they would ask a doctor new questions and change how they manage their health, chronic disease, or pain.	Not reported
Community Content Measures Outcomes	Randomized trial	Greater likelihood of intervention group to receive mammograms and Pap screening at 6-month follow-up. Also, increased HL and positive perception about cancer screening.	Effect sizes were large. After adjusting for covariates, the odds of participants receiving mammograms at 6 months were 18.5 times higher than for controls. The odds of participants getting Pap tests were 13.3 times higher than controls. Effect sizes were even higher when comparing intervention group participants who read all materials with those who did not.

continued

TABLE C-8 Continued

Author	Community	Setting	Topic	Intervention
Hansson and Markström 2014	Adults participating in police officer training at the University of Sweden	Police officer training sessions at university	Mental health	This study used a 3-week intervention to improve attitudes and MHL among police officers attending training at the University of Sweden. CAMI, MAKS, and RIBS.
Harrison, Ollis, and Savige 2016	Secondary school students	Schools in Geelong, Victoria, Australia	Student knowledge of and access to local health services; HL; help-seeking behaviors	Doc & Teens program delivered in schools by general practice doctors and teachers. HL survey used.
Hart, Berry, and Tonna 2011	People living in rural communities in New South Wales significantly impacted by drought	Neighborhood	Mental health	The purpose of this Rural Adversity Mental Health Services program was to disseminate information and organize community social events to raise MHL and analyze the effects of drought on mental health. Training was offered from 2007–2010, more than 3,000 people received it.

Health Literacy Component	Study Design	Outcomes	Magnitude
Measures Outcomes	Before–after study	Improved attitude, positivity about future interactions, and improved MHL as compared with comparison group.	Effect sizes for differences between intervention and control group increments immediately following the intervention were small to moderate for two attitude change items and for one intention to act item, and moderate for four MHL items. At 6 months following the intervention, the effect size was small for total attitudes and for intentions to work with mentally ill persons, and small to moderate for three MHL items.
Content Measures Outcomes	Other: Health curriculum using discussion and activities during school	Teachers and students rated the curriculum favorably, but little documented improvement in knowledge; mismatches in curriculum and what students wanted to learn.	Not reported
Content	Non-comparative study	Training of communities in MHFA; training of mental health workers to develop 15 local health, agriculture, and financial service networks; free mental health telephone line that took calls from 270 local farmers; multiple community events designed to raise awareness about drought-related mental health issues.	Not applicable

continued

TABLE C-8 Continued

Author	Community	Setting	Topic	Intervention
Hart, Jorm, and Paxton 2012	Undergraduate students living in residence halls at the University of Melbourne	University	Mental health, eating disorders	This single 4-hour classroom-style program was designed to provide Mental Health First Aid training to improve knowledge, behavior, and attitudes toward people with eating disorders. Used MHL Questionnaire for Bulimia Type Eating Disorders.
Hatamleh 2015	Adult Iraqi immigrants (18+) in the United States with English as a second language	Islamic community center in a large Midwestern city in the United States	HL skills (functional and complex)	Three-hour Arabic language educational program based on adult learning principles and topics identified through a community needs assessment (self-management; provider communication about medicines, tests, and forms). Used Test of All Aspects of Health Literacy Scale.

Health Literacy Component	Study Design	Outcomes	Magnitude
Content Measures Outcomes	Before–after study	No change in mean scores of knowledge of symptoms of eating disorders. Postintervention improvement found in problem recognition and knowledge of appropriate MHFA strategies ($p < 0.005$). The intervention had no effect on a measure of stigmatization nor on contact with persons experiencing eating disorders.	Not reported
Community Measures Content Outcomes	Before–after study	Average total HL score following intervention exceeded the pretest average ($p < 0.001$). This pattern was evident for communicative and critical HL subscales, but not for functional HL.	Not reported

continued

TABLE C-8 Continued

Author	Community	Setting	Topic	Intervention
Hernandez and Organista 2013	Latina immigrants at high risk for depression	Community center	Mental health	This study replicated the effectiveness of a Spanish-language fotonovela, a form of Entertainment–Education (E–E), designed to increase depression literacy, decrease stigma, and increase help-seeking knowledge and behavior in Latinas. Specifically, this study evaluated a fotonovela delivered in a multifaceted approach to health education used by promotoras. Used Short Test of Functional Health Literacy in Adults (S-TOFHLA).
Kim et al. 2014	Korean American older adults	Churches and senior centers in the Baltimore/ Washington, DC region	HBP	Community-based clinical trial to test the efficacy of a comprehensive management program to reduce blood pressure and increase HL. Six 2-hour sessions over 6 weeks. Used the HBP–Health Literacy Scale.

Health Literacy Component	Study Design	Outcomes	Magnitude
Community Content Measures Outcomes	Randomized trial	Results indicate significant posttest improvements in depression knowledge, SE to identify the need for treatment, and decreased stigma in experimental as compared with control group participants. Findings support the application of E–E health literacy tools such as fotonovelas, delivered in multifaceted approaches to health education used by promotoras, to Latinas at risk for mental health concerns.	Very large effect sizes emerged for the difference between intervention group members and controls in increments in (a) knowledge about depression and (b) SE to identify need for treatment. Effect size for differences in decrease in stigma and increase in intent to seek treatment were both moderate.
Community Content Measures Outcomes	Randomized trial	Participants in intervention group had better medication adherence; lower blood pressure; better HL scores at the 12- and 18-month follow-ups; more blood pressure knowledge; and less depression.	Not reported

continued

TABLE C-8 Continued

Author	Community	Setting	Topic	Intervention
Kim et al. 2015	Korean American adults with type 2 diabetes	Community center in Ellicott City, Maryland	Diabetes	Community-based, multimodal, behavioral self-help intervention program with six 2-hour in-class training sessions over 6 weeks to help first generation Korean American immigrants with diabetes achieve better glycemic control and restore their self-confidence in their diabetes management.
Lam 2014	Chinese middle-aged and older adults with diabetes	Diabetes centers in two hospitals in Hong Kong	Diabetes and physical activity	A nurse and certified exercise trainer led a 6-week group program using books and audiotapes to encourage participants to increase their physical activity. Six-week program with one 60-minute lesson a week at diabetes center. Used Chinese Health Literacy Scale for Diabetes.

Health Literacy Component	Study Design	Outcomes	Magnitude
Community Measures Content Outcomes	Randomized trial	Participants in HL-oriented program on physical activity behavior doubled their physical activity and attained acceptable levels.	Not reported
Content Measures Outcomes	Randomized trial	Participants in HL-oriented program on physical activity behavior doubled their physical activity from the sedentary to the internationally acceptable level.	Not reported

continued

TABLE C-8 Continued

Author	Community	Setting	Topic	Intervention
Lam, Jorm, and Wong 2010	Adult Chinese immigrants able to read and write basic Chinese	Recruited at social service agencies	Mental health	Impact of MHFA 12-hour training course on mental disorder knowledge and attitudes toward people with mental illness in a Chinese community in Melbourne. Instrument adapted for MHL.
Levin-Zamir et al. 2011	Ethiopian immigrants living in Israel	Community clinic	Health care access	Refuah Shlema program: Promote the health of the Ethiopian community via improved communication between primary care workers (physicians, nurses, pharmacists, and administrative staff) and immigrants based on the concepts of communication, advocacy, and HL.
Mahmud et al. 2010	30 "health squares" (collaborations between state-owned pharmacy and county councils)	Communities in Sweden	Health promotion and HL	Policy intervention to create new health promotion settings in communities and encourage individual responsibility.

Health Literacy Component	Study Design	Outcomes	Magnitude
Community Measures Outcomes	Before–after study	The intervention produced significant positive change in the level of MHL (at least $p < 0.05$) and reductions in stigmatizing attitudes ($p < 0.005$). There was no change from pre- to posttest in the belief that professional care would help someone experiencing depression or schizophrenia.	Not reported
Community	Other	Qualitative and quantitative evidence showed improvements in (1) clinic staff–patient relations; (2) availability and accessibility of health services and health system navigation without increasing service expenditure; (3) perception of general well-being; and (4) self-care practice regarding chronic conditions. Evidence significantly contributed to sustaining the program for 13+ years.	Not reported
Community	Policy analysis	Analysis of goals, activities, stakeholders, and factors affecting policy implementations showed intentions to use health squares for health promotion and HL, but did not share understanding of the concept.	Not applicable

continued

TABLE C-8 Continued

Author	Community	Setting	Topic	Intervention
Mancuso 2011	Indonesian refugee and asylum seekers	Health fair	Cardiovascular health and safe medicine use	Staff nurses and nursing and pharmacy students provided health checks and information on a range of health topics at a health fair.
Martin, Kripalani, and DuRapau 2012	Community-dwelling older adults in this study enrolled at an inner city adult day center who generally had low measured HL	Inner city adult day center	Medication adherence	Participants were given a personalized, illustrated daily medication schedule (PictureRx™). Six weeks later, their medication SE and adherence were assessed. NVS used.
Mindlis et al. 2015	People living in rural villages in India	Community center	Mental health and depression	This study compared knowledge and attitudes toward depression in villages where educational programs have targeted mental illness and stigma versus control villages. Series of interventions.

Health Literacy Component	Study Design	Outcomes	Magnitude
Community Content	Program evaluation via survey	Participant satisfaction with the health fair was positive.	Not reported
Community Measures Content Outcomes	Before–after study	Adherence to Refills and Medications Scale ($p < 0.05$) and SE for Appropriate Medication Use Scale ($p < 0.001$) scores improved after intervention.	Not reported
Community Measures Content Outcomes	Non-randomized trial, posttest only	Intervention villages showed higher levels of literacy regarding depression and lower levels of stigma, adjusting for sociodemographic variables.	Effect of residence in a treatment village was moderate.

continued

TABLE C-8 Continued

Author	Community	Setting	Topic	Intervention
Mosuro, Malcolm, and Guishard-Pine 2014	Foster caregivers in Great Britain	Training for foster caregivers	Mental health	This study examined the impact of a 30-hour counseling skills training course delivered over 3 months on foster caregivers' confidence in their counseling skills.
Muscat et al. 2016	Socially disadvantaged adults with low literacy	Adult education colleges in Australia	HL	Australian adaptation of U.K. Skilled for Health Program with content about managing health conditions and disease prevention/ health promotion embedded in literacy instruction. Eighty to 90 hours of instruction, either 8 hours/week for 10 weeks or 5 hours/ week for 18 weeks. Functional HL course-content–specific measure developed.
Noble, Hedmann, and Williams 2015	Elementary school students in Harlem, New York	Schools	Alzheimer's disease (AD) and dementia HL	In three 1-hour age-appropriate sessions over 3 consecutive days, the intervention used play, dance, and rap music to teach elementary school children to recognize AD symptoms and develop appropriate responses to them.

Health Literacy Component	Study Design	Outcomes	Magnitude
Community Content Measures Outcomes	Before–after study	Participants' confidence in their knowledge and understanding of the mental health needs of children in care increased after the intervention ($p < 0.01$). The intervention had no effect on caregivers' coping skills.	Not reported
Community Measures Content Outcomes	Cross-sectional study	Quantitative results showed improvements in participants' functional HL skills and confidence; very little change in mean total functional, critical, and communicative HL scores from baseline. Qualitative analysis identified positive student and teacher engagement with course content and self-reported improvements in health knowledge, attitudes, and communication with health care professionals.	Not reported
Content Measures Outcomes	Before–after study	Awareness of AD symptoms increased following the intervention and at delayed posttest ($p < 0.01$).	Not reported

continued

TABLE C-8 Continued

Author	Community	Setting	Topic	Intervention
Otilingam et al. 2015	Mexican-origin Latinas living in Los Angeles County	Clinic	Nutrition	Culturally tailored, theory-based nutrition education workshops taught in small groups included goal-setting and information about healthy eating. A second intervention arm provided information about brain health. Each workshop was 2 hours long. NVS used.
Oves 2013	Homeless mothers living in a residential rehabilitation facility in Atlanta, Georgia	Residential rehabilitation facility	Maternal and child health	A 6-hour maternal HL training to increase the health care knowledge of mothers who have been homeless.
Pais, Rodrigues, and Menezes 2014	School-aged adolescents	School and community organization	Formal and non-formal education for youth and children to promote HL	Study 2 presents four intensive case studies in schools where adolescents used community profiling, a participatory research methodology, to explore health rights and access to health care in both a historical and prospective vision.

Health Literacy Component	Study Design	Outcomes	Magnitude
Community Measures Content Outcomes	Randomized trial	Among those assigned to combined intervention arms, there was a statistically significant gain in HL ($p \leq 0.005$) and knowledge about dietary fat ($p < 0.05$). There was no pre- to posttest difference in outcomes for those given just the module about diet and brain health or for those in a control group.	Not reported
Community Measures Content Outcomes	Before–after study	Pre- to posttest shows training positively impacted reported maternal and child health knowledge; 2- to 4-month follow-up survey to 11% of the total sample showed women retained a considerable amount of knowledge.	Not reported
Content	Other	Community profiling projects regarded by pupils and teachers as meaningful learning experiences, with a positive impact on their sociopolitical development. Pupils increased knowledge about citizen health rights and the national health care system.	Not reported

continued

TABLE C-8 Continued

Author	Community	Setting	Topic	Intervention
Paul et al. 2015	Rural residents who use wells for water supply	Households in Tuftonboro, New Hampshire	Water contamination	Community presentations on water contamination and protective actions; community informational campaign; well water testing service for residents to make testing accessible and reduce inconvenience.
Pinto-Foltz, Logsdon, and Myers 2011	Females ages 13–17 in 9th and 10th grades in public high schools in southern urban area of the United States	Public high schools	MHL in adolescents	"In Our Own Voice" is a 60-minute program that was examined for feasibility, acceptability, and initial efficacy among female high school students in two southern U.S. schools. In Our Own Voice Knowledge Measure, developed by Wood and Wahl (2006).

Health Literacy Component	Study Design	Outcomes	Magnitude
Community	Other	Intended outcome was an increase in well water testing; after the intervention, state lab received more than triple the number of water tests than in prior 6 years.	Not reported
Community Measures Content Outcomes	Randomized trial	The intervention did not reduce mental illness stigma or improve MHL at 1-week follow-up. The intervention did not reduce mental illness stigma at 4- and 8-week follow-up. The intervention did improve MHL at 4- and 8-week follow-up.	Not reported

continued

TABLE C-8 Continued

Author	Community	Setting	Topic	Intervention
Pleasant 2011	Underserved communities	The Urban Health Plan is a federally qualified health center (FQHC)	Overall health, chronic disease	A program to increase HL and health behaviors among participants. Program was twice per week for 6 weeks.
Pomerantz et al. 2010	Working-class members of the community, especially disenfranchised people with little or no experience with the Internet and online health information resources	Community centers, libraries	Health information–seeking skills	Workshops on how to navigate the Internet, locate reliable health information online, and apply evaluation criteria. Two 3-hour Internet workshops.

Health Literacy Component	Study Design	Outcomes	Magnitude
Content Measures Outcomes	Other	Participants on average emerged from the program healthier in terms of physical and mental health. Participants experienced positive, statistically significant improvements in multiple indicators reflecting their physical health, fitness levels, self-reported health status, healthy behaviors, knowledge about health, attitudes toward their own ability to be healthy, amount of sleep, nutrition choices, and levels of stress and depression.	Not reported
Community Measures Outcomes	Before–after	Workshops showed modest improvement in posttest scores and postcards showed that people found the workshops interesting and helpful.	Not reported

continued

TABLE C-8 Continued

Author	Community	Setting	Topic	Intervention
Porter et al. 2016	Residents of eight rural southwest Virginia counties with documented health disparities (population is 48% female; 94% white; 42% high school education or less; average annual income is $48,104.27)	Classes in rural southwest Virginia (location of classes not reported)	Health behaviors, with focus on sugar-sweetened beverage consumption or physical activity	Classes, behavioral diaries, and a teach-back call to motivate and build skills for health behaviors, accurate completion of diaries, and personal action plans. This was a 6-month program. Used NVS.
Ramaswamy, Simmons, and Kelly 2015	English-speaking women over age 18 in a county jail in Kansas City, Kansas	Jail	Cervical cancer	The Sexual Health Empowerment (SHE) Project was a five-session, 2-hour cervical cancer education program implemented in a jail over 5 days. The goal was to increase cervical cancer knowledge, reduce barriers, and improve SE and confidence when navigating health systems. Used S-TOFHLA.

Health Literacy Component	Study Design	Outcomes	Magnitude
Community Measures Content Outcomes	Cross-sectional study	Participants with lower HL had lower accuracy with diary completion, recalled fewer behavior messages correctly, and required significantly more rounds of teach-back. There were outcome differences between participants in the beverage versus physical activity program.	Not reported
Community Content Measures Outcomes	Other	Increased confidence in navigating providers and health systems ($p = 0.02$). Changes in knowledge and SE were not statistically significant.	Not reported

continued

TABLE C-8 Continued

Author	Community	Setting	Topic	Intervention
Ramirez Andreotta et al. 2016	Predominately white, rural	Homes	Environmental health	Conducted interviews of families living on a Superfund site to determine whether communication materials that imparted knowledge of biometric results were effective and whether these efforts improved environmental HL.
Ramos et al. 2013	Hispanic males in rural areas of Shelbyville, Kentucky	Not listed	HL and disparities	Impact of culturally tailored health classes on the health knowledge of Hispanic residents of a rural town. Program had two phases, 2-hour sessions. HL assessment using standardized measures not completed, but HL indicators were used from Shelbyville Health Assessment.

Health Literacy Component	Study Design	Outcomes	Magnitude
Community Measures Outcomes	Cross-sectional study	In the interviews, participants reported implementing the exposure-reducing actions.	Not reported
Community Measures Content Outcomes	Before–after study	Improved performance scores in 100% of participants in Phase II. Overall knowledge: Participants scored 80% better on heart disease and stroke posttest, pretest knowledge of nutrition was low (20/25 scored below 50%), and overall posttest scores were 80%. 100% of participants showed improved scores in Phase II.	Not reported

continued

TABLE C-8 Continued

Author	Community	Setting	Topic	Intervention
Rodriguez 2015	Adult community college and night school class attendees (consisting of English- and/ or Spanish-speaking adults (n = 212; 91% Latino)	Schools	Dementia	This dissertation evaluated a dementia-themed fotonovela (graphic novel) to measure increase and maintenance of knowledge of dementia and improvement of SE and intention to help a family member with signs of dementia.
Romero et al. 2016	Hispanic women ages 18 to 85 with self-reported Spanish language preference and at least one or more self-reported risk factors for CVD, including HBP, high cholesterol, diabetes, excess weight, and/or smoking	Community center	CVD	This study adapted their own previously successful 12-week program into a 6-week course in Spanish to focus on CVD awareness among Hispanic women. Six-week program with one 90-minute session/week.

Health Literacy Component	Study Design	Outcomes	Magnitude
Community Content	Randomized trial	Groups who received dementia education via fotonovela or standard brochure showed improved knowledge compared with placebo. Fotonovela was not superior to brochure. Dementia knowledge increase maintained at 3-week follow-up in both groups compared with placebo. Not many differences between fotonovela and brochure in qualitative feedback, but the fotonovela was favored—participants found it easier and more enjoyable to read.	Not reported
Community Content	Before–after study	The mean CVD knowledge score for all participants increased from 39% to 66% postintervention. Completion of the program was associated with a 68% increase in overall mean CVD scores. There was a statistically significant increase in knowledge scores across all five CVD domains and a 57% increase in mean dietary knowledge score (43.7% [0 weeks], 68.7% [6 weeks], $p < 0.001$).	Not reported

continued

TABLE C-8 Continued

Author	Community	Setting	Topic	Intervention
Rubin et al. 2014	Meals on Wheels volunteers	Not listed	Aging	This intervention trained 73 Meals on Wheels volunteers to be HL coaches to reach a "hardly reached" population. Three- to 4-hour training workshops for coaches. One booster 1-hour session. Used S-TOFHLA.
Schuster et al. 2015	Korean American women overdue for mammograms and Pap tests	Church	Breast and cervical cancers	This paper aimed to determine the cost-effectiveness of an intervention. The intervention was aimed at increasing breast and cervical cancer screenings of Korean American women.
Shidhaye et al. 2017	Rural community members in India	Villages in India	Mental health	Vidarbha Stress and Health Programme (VISHRAM) was a multilayered community program based in rural India, aimed to address mental health and suicide.

Health Literacy Component	Study Design	Outcomes	Magnitude
Community Measures Content	Before–after study	Positive ratings for the workshop in self-reported learning, utility, quality of planning, and quality of workshop execution. Learned new information about communicating with older adults M = 6.63, SD = 1.09; increase on knowledge test from pretest to posttest was statistically significant (t70 = 3.57; $p < 0.001$). Does not give scores for improved HL.	Not reported
Community Content	Randomized trial	Cost-effectiveness ratio of intervention was estimated to be $236 per screening, without program development costs. This program offered a more cost-effective approach for promoting cancer screening.	Not reported
Community Measures Content Outcomes	Before–after study	Prevalence of current depression decreased from 14.6% to 11.3% at 18 months ($p = 0.005$). Contact coverage was six times higher at 18 months postsurvey, remaining after controlling for sociodemographics (4.3% to 27.2%, $p < 0.001$). Significant improvement in many MHL indicators. Most individuals with current depression sought care from general physicians, in line with the key message to seek help from these practitioners.	Not reported

continued

TABLE C-8 Continued

Author	Community	Setting	Topic	Intervention
Shreffler-Grant, Nichols, and Weinert 2017	Rural older adults	Senior citizen center in small rural community	HL	Program aimed to improve HL of older rural adults through complementary and alternative therapies. Sessions aimed to improve HL so participants could make more informed health decisions. Seven-week program, four sessions; sessions 1–1.5 hours long. NVS and single-item HL measure used.
Son et al. 2017	Incarcerated youth	Cuyahoga County Juvenile Detention Center	Reproductive health	An interactive 3-day curriculum was implemented in a juvenile detention center with the goal of increasing reproductive health knowledge and teachers' comfort level when teaching the topic.

Health Literacy Component	Study Design	Outcomes	Magnitude
Community Content Measures Outcomes	Before–after study	Increased comfort in using electronic sources to seek information, satisfaction with scheduling, and format of sessions other than webinars. Information on communicating with health care professionals helpful ($M = 4.63$ on 1–5 scale with 5 = definitely); increased comfort in using electronic sources to seek health info ($M = 4$). HL mean scores improved, but not statistically significant (pre: 70.3, post: 71.47, range 60–81); scale is 21 to 84.	Not reported
Community Measures Content Outcomes	Cohort	Increased knowledge regarding sexually transmitted infections and self-reported confidence in condom use ($p = 0.002$). SE in contraception use and sexual autonomy did not significantly improve.	Not reported

continued

TABLE C-8 Continued

Author	Community	Setting	Topic	Intervention
Soto Mas, Cordova, et al. 2015	Hispanic members of the Santa Barbara/ Martinez town community	Local elementary school (Site 1), large hotel chain (Site 2), and community church (Site 3)	HL	Study explored the feasibility of using different community settings for improving HL among adult Spanish speakers through an English-language program. The study used a pre-experimental, single-arm pre- and posttest design, and implemented the Health Literacy and ESL Curriculum. Curriculum is 12 units (approx. 45 min) implemented over 6 weeks. Spanish TOFHLA used.
Soto Mas, Ji, et al. 2015	Spanish-speaking adults living in El Paso, Texas	Three different community locations	HL	ESL instruction for improving HL among Spanish-speaking adults. Twelve units that can be implemented in 6 or 12 weeks. Used the TOFHLA.

Health Literacy Component	Study Design	Outcomes	Magnitude
Community Measures Content Outcomes	Before–after study	TOFHLA scores increased significantly in all sites; numeracy increased significantly in Sites 2 and 3; and reading comprehension significantly improved in Site 3. The Fisher's exact test based on the proposed level change index yielded a non-statistically significant association among sites and a change in HL level.	Not reported
Community Measures Content Outcomes	Randomized trial	Intervention participants had a significant average change score on TOFHLA after intervention ($p < 0.01$). Percentage of intervention participants at inadequate functional HL level decreased at posttest by 30% and adequate functional HL increased by 24%. Control group percentage at the inadequate functional HL level decreased at posttest by 11% and adequate functional HL increased by 21%.	Not reported

continued

TABLE C-8 Continued

Author	Community	Setting	Topic	Intervention
Stockwell et al. 2010	Latino EHS parents in Washington Heights, New York	University-affiliated EHS in New York City	Upper respiratory infections	This intervention aimed to increase HL regarding upper respiratory infections because of treatment misconceptions, especially in the Latino community. Used Knowledge, Attitudes, Practices (KAP) instrument.
Svensson Hansson, and Stjernswärd 2015	Western and northern Sweden; diverse organizations and occupational groups represented	Premises booked by the local coordinators in six cities	Mental Health First Aid	This was a qualitative study using participants in Sweden to explore the effects of Mental Health First Aid on participants. Training is a 12-hour course.
Taylor et al. 2012	Aboriginal Australian community members	Three Aboriginal communities in Australia	Dementia	This study piloted a dementia education program (16-minute DVD) in English and in three Aboriginal languages.

Health Literacy Component	Study Design	Outcomes	Magnitude
Community Content Measures Outcomes	Before–after study	Increased knowledge, attitudes, and HL. Positive change in care practices and decreased incorrect medication usage.	Not reported
Content	Qualitative analysis of participants' responses to training	Participants found the program practical, regardless of their professional orientation and experience. Participation in the course, for people with mixed experience of meeting those with mental health issues, appears to contribute to an increased confidence and inclination to act when meeting a person suspected of having mental health problems.	Not applicable
Community Content	Qualitative analysis of focus group responses	Resource was effective in raising awareness of dementia as a health issue for remote Indigenous communities. Qualitative work identified elements that helped or hindered the communication of the dementia education message.	Not applicable

continued

TABLE C-8 Continued

Author	Community	Setting	Topic	Intervention
Tuerk et al. 2013	Residents of Mito, Japan, area hit by a devastating earthquake	Community auditorium	Posttraumatic stress, mental health	Trainings were held to address posttraumatic stress after an earthquake in Japan. Questionnaires were distributed and integrated into the training to increase MHL. Training was 2.5 hours.
Unger et al. 2013	Southern California Hispanic community	Community adult school, Los Angeles Unified School District	Depression	Participants randomized to fotonovela or National Institutes of Health (NIH) low-literacy text pamphlet about depression, with the goal of increased long-term depression knowledge and dissemination of information through social networks. Thirty minutes with either fotonovela or pamphlet.

Health Literacy Component	Study Design	Outcomes	Magnitude
Community Content Measures Outcomes	Postevent survey	27% met criteria for probable posttraumatic stress disorder (PTSD), with 15% reporting that the recent earthquake was the index event. Intervention yielded positive screening rates of 8% for probable PTSD and 4% for probable PTSD related to earthquake. Physical health problems increased in the past 7 days and loss of sense of community related to PTSD symptoms, after controlling for covariates.	Not reported
Community Content	Randomized trial	Increased depression knowledge in both groups $p < 0.05$, retained at 1 month, but decreased. Knowledge increase significantly larger for fotonovela at post ($p < 0.05$), but not follow-up. Antidepressant stigma decreased in fotonovela, not in comparison group ($p < 0.05$), follow-up regressed to pretest. Mental health care stigma decreased in fotonovela ($p < 0.05$), not in comparison group; further decreased at follow-up ($p < 0.05$). SE increased in both groups and remained significant at follow-up ($p < 0.05$). When seeking help, both groups experienced ceiling effect, no differences. Fotonovelas were more likely to be shared and not thrown away ($p < 0.01$).	Not reported

continued

TABLE C-8 Continued

Author	Community	Setting	Topic	Intervention
Vanderbilt et al. 2016	Participants were required to be over the age of 18, pass the computer skills test with a 70% or higher, and live in the Richmond-Metro area community serviced by one of the resource centers	Resource centers in participants' communities	eHealth Literacy, preterm birth HL	This computer-based intervention sought to increase HL regarding preterm birth. Five computer-based educational modules, approximately 1 hour each.
Vollmer Dahlke et al. 2017	Adolescent and young adult (AYA) cancer survivors ("participants were clinicians, AYA cancer survivors, caregivers, and cancer advocates affiliated with the Seton Healthcare Family in Austin, Texas")	Medical practices and hospitals	Cancer	This qualitative study provided assessment of a cancer literacy program aimed at increasing HL among adolescent and young adult cancer survivors and their health care providers. Two annual half-day interactive educational sessions.

Health Literacy Component	Study Design	Outcomes	Magnitude
Community Content Measures Outcomes	Before–after study	Increased knowledge in HL and preterm birth. Findings suggest that computer-based modules developed (intervention) to educate adults in an underserved community about preterm birth and HL have the potential to decrease health disparities.	Not reported
Community Measures Content Outcomes	Other	Evaluation results highlight the need to continue to build both survivor and professional resources to address the unique impact of cancer on AYA cancer survivors.	Not reported

continued

TABLE C-8 Continued

Author	Community	Setting	Topic	Intervention
White et al. 2012	People taking self-care skills training courses in parent and child groups and in workplaces within intervention Primary Care Trusts	Non-clinical settings	Self-care	This 12-month study evaluated a self-care skills training course (Self Care for People) within workplace and parent and toddler group settings. The course was six 3-hour sessions over a 3- to 6-week period. This study did not attempt to change health behavior, and states that it is policy driven. Primary outcome: change in number of general practitioner (GP) consultations between baseline and follow-up. HL scale developed by research team.
Wong et al. 2017	Ages 18+ with ability to understand Chinese	Not specified	Mental health	This study presented a 12-hour MHFA course with the aim of increasing mental health recognition knowledge and reducing stigma among participants. Used MHL scale.

Health Literacy Component	Study Design	Outcomes	Magnitude
Measures Outcomes	Before–after study	No change in use of GP services. Increased use of out-of-hours and secondary care services. At 6-month follow-up, statistically significant small positive effects on self-esteem, well-being, and anxiety scores for intervention group. At 12-month follow-up, statistically significant small positive effects seen on recovery locus of control, HL, and self-esteem scores, and on knowledge of adult cough for intervention group.	The intervention effect size was small for using services in the follow-up period; for using out-of-hour services; and for outpatient visits. The effect on hospital admissions was small to moderate.
Community Measures Outcomes	Non-randomized trial	Participants who received training in MHFA progressed from pretest to posttest on MHL items, destigmatization, and efficacy in offering help. The same pattern was found for the delayed posttest, except for two MHL items. While treatment groups were equivalent at pretest, at posttest and delayed posttest the MHFA group exceeded the control, except for two MHL items.	Effect sizes were small for differences between pretest and posttest, and differences between pretest and posttest scores on MHL, efficacy for helping, and destigmatization, except for moderate effect sizes for pretest to posttest changes in two MHL items.

continued

TABLE C-8 Continued

Author	Community	Setting	Topic	Intervention
Xie 2011	Adults ages 60–89	Public libraries	E-health literacy in older adults	This study was a 4-week, two times per week, 2-hour course that trained participants on how to use a computer, the Internet, and how to navigate two NIH websites to improve adult (age 60+) access to and use of high-quality health information on the Internet.
Zhuang et al. 2016	Adults ages 18+ living in Shenzhen, China	Cell phone	HL	This study explored using SMS (text) messages to deliver health education and aimed to improve the HL of a community in China. Intervention group received conventional health education measures and health education messages once per week for 1 year. Used REALM.

NOTES: Chan 2012, refers to a single dissertation with two studies. BC = breast cancer; CAMI = Community Attitudes toward the Mentally Ill Scale; CHW = community health worker; CVD = cardiovascular diseases; E–E = entertainment–education; EHS = Early Head Start; ESL = English as a second language; GP = general practitioner; HBP = high blood pressure; HL = health literacy; HLQ = Health Literacy Questionnaire; IDA = iron-deficiency anemia; MAKS = Mental Health Knowledge Scale; MHFA = mental health first aid; MHL = mental health literacy; NGO = nongovernmental organization; NIH = National Institutes of Health; NVS = Newest Vital Sign; REALM = Rapid Assessment of Adult Literacy in Medicine; RIBS = Reported and Intended Behavior Scale; SE = self-efficacy; SES = socioeconomic status; SNAP = Supplemental Nutrition Assistance Program; S-TOFHLA = Short Test of Functional Health Literacy in Adults; YMCA = Young Men's Christian Association.

Health Literacy Component	Study Design	Outcomes	Magnitude
Community Content Measures Outcomes	Before–after study	All hypotheses were supported, except H4. Dependent t-tests indicated that computer anxiety significantly decreased from pre- to postintervention, while computer interest and efficacy significantly increased. Participants (78%) reported that what they learned from the training had affected their participation in their own health care.	Not reported
Community Measures Content Outcomes	Before–after study	Public HL scores increased 1.5 points, from 61.8 to 63.3, after SMS intervention for 1 year ($p < 0.01$); increase greater for males than females ($p < 0.01$); frequency of high HL scores was greater for the intervention than control group (22.03% to 30.93% versus 22.07% to 20.82%).	Not reported

TABLE C-9 Frequency of Labels to Identify Intervention Communities

Groups	Number of Articles*
Asian	N = 15
Hispanic/Latino	N = 11
Rural	N = 9
School-aged children/Youth	N = 8
Community health workers/Health coaches	N = 5
Immigrants	N = 6
Older adults	N = 6
Parents	N = 6
African American	N = 3

*Based on N = 74 papers, but column will not total 74 because articles could be in more than one category, and not all communities in the 74 papers are listed in the table.

discussed below in the culturally sensitive interventions category. Most of these interventions occurred in countries other than those in North America and Western Europe. An intervention in Pakistan had a two-part purpose of increasing female college students' communication skills and sense of civic responsibility and increasing the iron-deficiency anemia knowledge of local women in a vocational education program (Ayub et al. 2015). The researchers described their program as a health literacy intervention because they aimed to create a trained, volunteer public health workforce to help meet the needs of low-literacy communities and build health knowledge. The researchers used pre- and posttests to identify statistically significant increases in students' perception of civic responsibility; students' perception of communication competency; and community women's knowledge of iron-deficiency anemia. Notably, the least educated community women showed the lowest knowledge gain.

The review identified several papers featuring the Ophelia (OPtimising Health LiterAcy and Access) approach developed by Richard Osborne and colleagues in Australia. A summary paper that reports intervention results from nine diverse sites in Australia met the inclusion criteria (Beauchamp et al. 2017). Readers can refer to the Ophelia protocol (Batterham et al. 2014), a Health Literacy Questionnaire validation study (Elsworth, Beauchamp, and Osborne 2016), and a detailed report of one of the nine sites (Goeman et al. 2016) (see results in Table C-8 for Goeman et al.) to learn more about the Ophelia model. The purpose of the nine interventions was to demonstrate "the successful application of the eight underlying principles to achieve development of health-literacy informed interventions with the potential to impact health and health outcomes" (Beauchamp et al. 2017, 5). Each site had a primary service organization that led the project and defined its own intervention outcomes based on their clients' responses to the Health Literacy Questionnaire, a survey instrument designed and validated by the research team. In general, the intended outcomes were improving clients' health literacy or identifying ways to make information or services more accessible. The authors report that of the six sites that used the Health Literacy Questionnaire to measure intervention outcomes, four found effects ranging mainly from small to moderate. Qualitative evaluation methods found a range of improvements that included self-efficacy, communication with providers, information seeking, and applying what was learned. Sites that involved volunteers reported they felt involved and useful in helping others.

A research team in the United Kingdom implemented an existing program called Self Care for People with the aim of increasing participants' self-care knowledge and skills and their confidence and intention to do self-care (White et al. 2012). The primary outcome was a change in the number of general practitioner consultations between baseline and follow-up over a 12-month period. The self-care program consisted of six three-hour sessions over a 3- to 6-week period. Participants received a handbook and exercises. The classes were held in small group sessions in workplaces and community-service locations for parents. Comparing the intervention groups to similar locations used as controls, the team did not find a significant difference in the use of general practitioner services after the self-care program. At the 6- and 12-month follow-ups, the researchers did find small but statistically significant improvements in intermediate outcomes, such as self-esteem and health literacy, defined as decisions about when to use services, intention to use services, and exposure to other self-care initiatives and resources.

In Shenzhen, China, a research team sampled communities by streets and residential buildings to be part of a health literacy intervention or control group (Zhuang et al. 2016). Both groups received basic health education through bulletin boards, posters, and health lectures; the intervention group also received text messages once a week for 1 year. The health content consisted of data, explanations, and recommended health behaviors encouraging action. Using a pre/post 22-item questionnaire with dimensions of health knowledge, behavior, and skill, researchers found that the intervention group had slightly higher health literacy scores after 1 year than the control group. The researchers also analyzed the acceptability of receiving messages and cost-effectiveness.

A research team in Georgia partnered with Meals on Wheels, a volunteer organization that delivers meals daily to homebound older adults. The team trained the volunteer drivers to deliver a health literacy skills intervention to the older adults they visited (Rubin et al. 2014). The intervention adapted a 2002 Meals on Wheels program used in southern Oregon as well as *Questions Are the Answer* (AHRQ) and the *AskMe3* campaign (National Patient Safety Foundation). The volunteers scored near the top of the range on the Short Test of Functional Health Literacy for Adults, and their assignment was to foster interactive health literacy skills with the older adult clients so they could communicate more effectively with their health care providers. The paper reported the results of the training workshop and clients' recall of the coaching they received. The volunteers scored the workshops as effective, and client recall of the coaching interventions was high. Using a sample of clients who received the coaching and were contacted in the twelve months following, 93 percent recalled the coaching events; 83 percent said they thought about "good questions for good health"; and more than 75 percent could recall a specific coaching practice.

One study interested in people's self-monitoring skills used a group class on either sugar-sweetened beverage consumption or physical activity, behavioral diaries, and a teach-back call to assess people's accuracy in recalling messages and behaviors (Porter et al. 2016). The researchers measured participants' baseline health literacy with the Newest Vital Sign (Weiss et al. 2005). The researchers were interested in participants' ability to accurately complete food diaries and recall behavioral messages, as well as the amount of teach-back needed to confirm understanding. They found that overall, participants with the lowest levels of health literacy had the greatest difficulties with accuracy and recall and needed more teach-back. Compared to those who received the sugar-sweetened beverage content, the participants in the physical activity arm more accurately completed their diaries, but recalled fewer behavioral messages and needed more teach-back (Porter et al. 2016).

An academic–community partnership on Long Island, New York, used health literacy content in a miniature public health curriculum for community residents (Goodman, Dias, and Stafford 2010). The goal was to bridge cultural divides and increase residents' "science" and "research" literacy so that they could participate in a community health collaborative. Residents asked for the training so that they would be on "equal footing" with researchers. The curriculum consisted of eleven didactic sessions and four experiential workshops; sessions were held at public libraries because they were accessible and trusted local spaces. Adult literacy instructors helped to develop the curriculum. Outcome measures were knowledge change; participant satisfaction; and submission of a pilot grant proposal to the university partner. Pre- and posttests showed improved knowledge of public health research topics, and open-ended questions elicited positive responses to the curriculum with requests for more time spent on content and group activities. Ten of the thirteen community members in the sessions submitted pilot grant proposals.

Information-Seeking Interventions

Three projects focused on improving people's health information-seeking skills. In Australia, a team of clinicians, consumer representatives, and librarians led free public workshops to help adults improve their online skills in finding and using evidence-based health information (Gray, Elliott, and Wale 2013). Workshop participants were overwhelmingly positive about the workshops' effects on knowledge, skills, attitudes, and potential impact on seeking behaviors. Participants also reported that they intended to ask doctors new questions and change how they maintained their health and coped with chronic disease and pain. Higher income and being native born were associated with more positive reports about the workshops' impact. A similar intervention for working-class community members in the Washington, DC, area also found modest improvements in participants' ability to find and evaluate online information (Pomerantz et al. 2010). A computer skills and health information-seeking improvement intervention in suburban Maryland targeted older adults (Xie 2011). The research team offered public library-based classes using materials from the National Institute on Aging to help older adults learn how to use MedlinePlus.gov and NIHSeniorHealth.gov. Pre- and posttests showed significant improvements in computer and Web knowledge, along with decreased anxiety, increased efficacy, and increased participation in health care.

Culturally Sensitive Interventions to Build Knowledge and Skills

Five interventions aimed to increase not only health knowledge, but also behaviors and skills, such as communicating with others about health, seeking information, asking questions, and analyzing information, for distinct cultural groups; more interventions targeting cultural groups are discussed in the adult learners, chronic disease, mental health (other), and cancer sections. A project in a Midwestern U.S. city aimed to improve the functional, communicative, and critical health literacy skills of Iraqi immigrants for whom English is a second language (Hatamleh 2015). Using feedback from a community needs assessment, the researcher developed a three-hour educational session in Arabic that covered all types of health literacy skills and used a pre- and posttest to examine the effects. Functional health literacy (understanding information; familiarity with available resources; and ability to complete forms) did not improve as much as participants' self-reported ability to communicate with providers and critically assess information.

A 13-year program in Israel aimed to assist Ethiopian immigrants and improve their health by providing educational sessions and cultural liaisons and helping them communicate with health care workers (Levin-Zamir et al. 2011). The intervention also trained clinic staff to bridge cultural differences. The researchers reported improvements in clinic–patient relations; availability and accessibility of health services; improved navigation; and perceived well-being and self-management.

A health literacy model of behavior change was designed to help adults improve specific mental and physical health behaviors (Pleasant 2011). Facilitators varied in professional background and included physicians, nurses, nutritionists, physical therapists, social workers, and a pastor. Participants were recruited from a federally qualified community health center. Sessions were hosted in English and Spanish and held twice per week over a 6-week period. Interactive sessions employed lectures, activity, and goal setting. A few of the positive health changes include improved health values (cholesterol, blood pressure), increased exercise, improved nutrition, and increased physical ability. Additionally, participants reported changes in behaviors and attitudes, as well as gains in health literacy, such as reading and understanding food labels.

Two interventions for Indonesian refugees and asylum seekers in New Hampshire focused on explaining safe medicine use, empowering individuals to understand and access the health care system, and improving communication with health care providers (Mancuso 2011). One intervention was a community program on safe medicine use and provided a lecture, question-and-answer session, brochures, and wallet cards. A second intervention was a health fair with prevention information; body mass index, blood pressure, and cholesterol checks; instruction on how to read a food label; brown-bag medicine check-ups; and referrals to local care providers. Organizers received positive evaluations from community participants and health professionals.

Adult Learners and Health Literacy Interventions

A subset of health literacy knowledge and skill improvement interventions focused on adult learners. Several projects examined the effects of integrating health literacy content in adult education programs (Brown, Collie-Akers, and Fernandez-Ortega 2015; Chervin et al. 2012; Freedman 2011; Muscat et al. 2016; Soto Mas, Cordova, et al. 2015; Soto Mas, Ji, et al. 2015). As Soto Mas and two sets of colleagues (Soto Mas, Cordova, et al. 2015; Soto Mas, Ji, et al. 2015) observed, the *National Action Plan to Improve Health Literacy* (HHS 2010) calls for the integration of adult literacy curricula and health literacy content, but few examples exist of how to combine them. In one project, six adult education centers in the North-east United States used a "study circles" approach to train adult education teachers to teach health literacy skills and integrate health literacy content into the curriculum (Rudd et al. 2005; cited in Chervin et al. 2012). The project goal was not only to improve adult learners' health literacy skills and increase their self-efficacy, but also to show how to teach health literacy as part of adult education. An evaluation found students' knowledge about health issues and self-efficacy increased significantly as a result of the health literacy instruction, and all six centers improved their capacity to teach health literacy. A knowledge and self-efficacy building intervention for primarily Latino adults attending adult community college or night school classes also found knowledge increases using either a fotonovela or brochure (Rodriguez 2015). A case study of a health literacy skills class in Atlanta, Georgia, described the effects of teaching functional health literacy skills to adult learners (Freedman 2011). The researcher was interested in how health literacy instruction could help adult learners to take greater control of their health and use what they learned in everyday life. She found that "careful attention to environmental factors and instructional strategies" can improve learning and help students carry lessons into everyday health behavior change (Freedman 2011, 81).

Five interventions conducted in English-speaking countries specifically considered the issues of health literacy for non-native speakers of English (Brown, Collie-Akers, and Fernandez-Ortega 2015; Muscat et al. 2016; Otilingam et al. 2015; Soto Mas, Cordova, et al. 2015; Soto Mas, Ji, et al. 2015). Soto Mas and colleagues implemented their Health Literacy and ESL (English as a second language) Curriculum with native Spanish speakers in two different U.S. communities to see if they could improve participants' health literacy as measured by the Test of Functional Health Literacy in Adults (TOFHLA) (Soto Mas, Cordova, et al. 2015; Soto Mas, Ji, et al. 2015). The Health Literacy and ESL Curriculum is a 12-unit package that includes traditional grammar, vocabulary, reading, writing, speaking, civic and life skills, math, and two health units. Certified ESL instructors teach the curriculum in 6 or 12 weeks. A 6-week implementation in New Mexico used a local elementary school, large hotel chain (employer), and community church as classroom sites. Using the Spanish version, the research team found that total TOFHLA, raw numeracy, and reading comprehension scores increased significantly; only two participants scored inadequate functional health literacy at posttest compared with thirteen at baseline (Soto Mas, Cordova, et al. 2015). Using a control group and the English-language TOFHLA to measure health literacy, a 6-week implementation in Texas significantly increased the intervention group's TOFHLA score compared with a control group (Soto Mas, Ji, et al. 2015).

Two interventions focused on nutrition topics and Spanish-speaking Latinas of Mexican origin (Brown, Collie-Akers, and Fernandez-Ortega

2015; Otilingam et al. 2015; see also Castañeda et al. 2016 in the cancer section). A nutrition literacy project used the SNAP-ED program, a federal program to reduce food insecurity and improve nutrition and wellness of low-resource groups, to reach Spanish-speaking women with low literacy skills (Brown, Collie-Akers, and Fernandez-Ortega 2015). The researchers tried the intervention with SNAP-ED clients as well as bilingual peer educators. The clients chose MyPyramid, reading Nutrition Facts labels, and using portion control for meals as the skills they wanted to learn. A qualitative evaluation found that participants rated the workshop and curriculum "very useful." Otilingam and colleagues (2015) developed and tested *Buenos Hábitos Alimenticios para Una Buena Salud*, a program of two 2-hour nutrition workshops for Latinas. The workshops had culturally relevant nutrition information and skill-building activities, such as reading Nutrition Facts labels and preparing low-fat meals. The workshops were held in a community clinic familiar to workshop participants. Researchers used the Newest Vital Sign as a health literacy pre- and post-test and measured knowledge and self-reported health behaviors (Weiss et al. 2005). Compared with control groups, intervention groups showed health literacy, knowledge, and self-reported behavior improvements. Participants said the most important thing they learned was how to read nutrition labels.

An Australian project adapted a U.K. adult and health literacy program and conducted a feasibility study of an integrated adult and health literacy curriculum to improve functional, communicative, and critical health literacy skills (Muscat et al. 2016). The study mainly enrolled culturally and linguistically diverse students who spoke a language other than English. The students reported being satisfied and engaged with the content and said they were better prepared to communicate with health care professionals, including asking questions. However, the results of the evaluation questionnaires showed improvements in topic-specific health literacy, but no significant improvement in a composite measure of generic functional, communicative, and critical health literacy skills (Muscat et al. 2016).

Early Childhood Education and Health Literacy Interventions

The review includes three articles that involved Head Start programs, parents, or children (Burgette 2016; Fleary 2012; Stockwell et al. 2010). One project aimed to improve community members' oral health through a health literacy intervention. The project focused on training Early Head Start teachers and staff so they could educate parents and children less than three years old about good oral health and prevention, especially during pregnancy and for infants and young children (Burgette 2016). The educational intervention was Zero Out Early Childhood Caries. Baseline and

24-month reports indicated that children enrolled in this program were more likely to have had a dental visit and less likely to have negative quality of life results than children in the Medicaid control group. Parents' health literacy was not a significant factor for the Head Start children's results. A second intervention recruited mothers with children in a Texas Head Start program to participate in a 5-week educational intervention about healthy lifestyles, including diet/nutrition, physical activity, sleep hygiene, parenting skills, and mental wellness (Fleary 2012); the mothers' knowledge about all topics increased. In New York City, researchers partnered with adult literacy experts to create a culturally appropriate educational program in English and Spanish and care kit for upper respiratory infections, based on CDC campaign materials (Stockwell et al. 2010). The purpose was to educate low-income Latino parents with children in Early Head Start programs about appropriate care for upper respiratory infections. Researchers reported that parents' knowledge increased, and parents' attitudes about appropriate care changed.

Schools as Health Literacy Intervention Sites

This section reports on four studies that used schools as the setting for health literacy interventions; three additional school-based and one university-based study are reported in the mental health section (Fung et al. 2016; Hart, Jorm, and Paxton 2012; Noble, Hedmann, and Williams 2015; Pinto-Foltz, Logsdon, and Myers 2011), and one additional school-based study is reported in the medicine section (Chang et al. 2015). An intervention in Spain and one in Portugal tried to change student, school, and community engagement for health improvement. One project examined how schools in low-income, immigrant communities in Spain could use family-oriented health programs to reduce inequalities and foster social inclusion (Flecha, García, and Rudd 2011). Using a case study evaluation approach, the researchers found that the schools that paid close attention to a community's expressed needs, created a welcoming space for community members to gather, and included the community's "cultural intelligence" or rich knowledge about their own experience and needs were the most successful in addressing the community's health literacy needs and improving adults' and children's health literacy. Pais and colleagues (2014) worked with high school students to enhance health literacy through a community profiling project. Students assessed community needs and resources and took a leadership role in working with community members, professionals, and political representatives to address identified needs. The authors present two case studies from secondary schools in Porto, Portugal. Students negotiated topics with their teachers and workgroups and selected examination of health rights and health care service costs. Students participated in every phase of the research, created poster presentations, and discussed findings at a symposium at the University of Porto. Students said they valued the opportunity to share and listen to varied opinions during the poster symposium. Teachers observed students' increased ability to make critical judgments about past and present situations. The authors suggest the students' experience helped them exercise their citizenship, thus developing a foundation for critical health literacy in the future.

Diamond and colleagues (2011) used the Building Wellness Curriculum to design an after-school program for third through eighth grade students. Students came from urban communities, had high risk for chronic disease, and qualified for no-cost school lunches. Topics included food choices, healthy choices, body function, and skills about communicating with a health provider. The course was offered for one semester during each academic year over a span of 6 years and used discussion, in-class activities, reflection, and take-home activities. Researchers used the REALM Teen program to assess health literacy at years one, three, and six. Findings suggested consistent increases in knowledge and retention of information. Teachers' anecdotal reports indicate students demonstrated positive behavior changes and increased curiosity about health and the body. By contrast, a school-based project in Australia used general practice doctors and teachers to lead a health curriculum to increase high school students' health literacy, help-seeking behaviors, and access to local health services (Harrison, Ollis, and Savige 2016). Researchers found the students were receptive to the doctors and teachers as health resources, but the volume of information was overwhelming and not sufficiently in-depth on key topics. The evaluation found that even though students could recall information, there was little improvement in student knowledge, confidence, help-seeking behavior, or ability or desire to access health services.

Other Settings or Topics for Health Literacy Interventions

Son and colleagues (2016) worked with health care students to facilitate a three-day curriculum about "reproductive health literacy" at a juvenile detention center (see the cancer section for an additional study with incarcerated women) (Ramaswamy, Simmons, and Kelly 2015). The authors described "reproductive health literacy" as knowledge, self-efficacy, and communication skills. Participants were female and averaged age 16 years. Study findings were increased knowledge about sexually transmitted infections and increased self-efficacy in condom use. However, there was no significant improvement in sexual autonomy or contraception use.

Adult residents of the Richmond, Virginia, metropolitan area participated in a computer-based intervention to increase health literacy about preterm births (Vanderbilt et al. 2016). The majority (95 percent) of participants were African-American; about 20 percent of participants were male. Six modules included information about preterm births and related risk factors. The researchers said the modules used adult learning theory and plain language, among other techniques, to make the content accessible; the modules were reviewed by a range of experts, including health literacy experts. Women showed significant knowledge gains for all six modules. However, men did not show significant increases for the modules *Let's Talk Patient and Provider Communication* and *It Takes a Village*.

An intervention in Atlanta, Georgia, aimed to improve maternal and child health outcomes by building the knowledge of mothers who were homeless, had addiction problems, and lived in a rehabilitation facility (Oves 2013). Information for the mothers pertained to newborn care, preventive services, and social services. The mothers participated in a 6-hour class and received a manual. Using pre- and posttests, the researcher found increases in knowledge after the class and in a subsample at 2 to 4 months post-intervention.

Chronic Disease Risks and Management

Eight interventions focused on low health literacy adult groups with respect to chronic disease risk reduction and disease self-management. The interventions integrated health literacy techniques, such as simplified content and easy, action-oriented recommendations, to improve health literacy and sometimes change behavioral or physiological outcomes related to diabetes and cardiovascular risks or disease.

Chan's (2012) dissertation research in Hong Kong included two studies of older Chinese adults (average age 73 years) with one or more chronic diseases; the researcher chose older adults with chronic diseases because the literature review identified older adults as having low health literacy. To improve their health literacy as well as other outcomes, one study examined the effects of multiple-exposure, group self-management classes on self-management behaviors; self-efficacy; health status; and health care use (Chan 2012). Chan's interventions used simplified content, including plain Chinese and concrete examples. Using an intervention and control group, the researcher found statistically significant improvements in all self-management behaviors and self-efficacy outcomes and half of the health status measures. No change in health care use was found. In the second study (Chan 2012), the researcher proposed that well-designed diabetes self-management programs could improve adherence, health literacy, and health outcomes (Chan 2012, 16). The plain Chinese-language intervention included multiple-exposure, group diabetes educational sessions designed to improve a range of outcomes, including knowledge, quality of life, mental health, food consumption, and physiological measures. Using an intervention and control group, the researcher found statistically significant improvements in diabetes-related knowledge and quality of life, along with reductions in total energy and saturated fat intake. No changes in physiological measures, such as blood sugar and blood pressure levels, or other nutritional and quality-of-life measures were found.

Lam (2014) also conducted an intervention with Chinese adults (45 years and older) in Hong Kong, again because of their low health literacy and its relation to chronic disease management; the purpose was to increase their physical activity and improve their diabetes outcomes. Lam describes the intervention as culture, language, disease, and age appropriate, as well as theory based and "health literacy-oriented," meaning the intervention was "a patient self-care empowerment program to nurture patients' ability to obtain, understand, comprehend, and analyze the health information and services that they needed [sic]" (Lam 2014, 18). A nurse and certified exercise trainer led the six-week classes followed by a telephone follow-up. Compared with the control group that received standard diabetes education, the intervention participants doubled their physical activity levels from sedentary to acceptable levels; no health literacy results were reported.

Two different interventions targeted Korean Americans with chronic conditions (Kim et al. 2014; Kim et al. 2015). One focused on older adults (average age 70 years) with high blood pressure who were selected because of low health literacy (Kim et al. 2014). A high blood pressure management intervention for Korean-American older adults added a health literacy component to educate participants about words and phrases relevant to blood pressure as well as communication skills with providers (Kim et al. 2014). The team used a high blood pressure health literacy scale they had validated in other research. The intervention was delivered in small groups at churches and senior centers over 6 weeks. In comparison to the control group, the intervention group had better medication adherence; lower blood pressure; better health literacy scores at the 12- and 18-month follow-ups (but not the 6-month follow-up); more blood pressure knowledge; and less depression. In the other study with first generation Korean-American immigrant adults (35 years or older), researchers selected the participants because of low health literacy and reported problems even using health materials in their native language (Kim et al. 2015). The health literacy component focused on building skills for tasks such as reading food labels and understanding medical terms; this was done through 2-hour group education sessions over 6 weeks. Although the researchers identified health literacy as a secondary outcome, it was not measured and reported separately in the results. The researchers found the intervention group improved on all outcomes of hemoglobin A1c levels, diabetes-related knowledge and self-efficacy, and quality of life in comparison with the control group (Kim et al. 2015).

An intervention on diabetes and blood pressure knowledge and self-efficacy involved older African Americans (average age 72 years) with low health literacy in senior affordable housing complexes in Washington, DC, and Maryland (Bertera 2014). The researcher designed and tested educational materials featuring community members as "talent"; combined the African American tradition of oral storytelling with the Hispanic medium of fotonovelas; and provided group educational sessions. Using intervention and control groups and pre- and posttests, the researcher showed a statistically significant increase in intervention participants' knowledge and self-efficacy. Using Chew et al.'s (2008) item set, the researcher found intervention participants with the lowest scores reported the greatest gains in self-efficacy.

Two interventions were implemented with Hispanic community members (see the culturally sensitive interventions, adult learners, mental health [other], and cancer sections for more interventions with Hispanic/Latino community members). Using data from a community health needs assessment and feedback from community leaders, a team in Shelbyville, Kentucky, created an educational program, "The Environment and Your Health" (Ramos et al. 2013). The curriculum placed special emphasis on cardiovascular disease and diabetes. Hispanic residents took two sets of health topic-specific classes 9 months apart, and pre- and posttests showed significant knowledge gains. In Boston, Massachusetts, researchers adapted a successful cardiovascular risk reduction program for African American women (Love Your Heart) and low-income Hispanic women (Romero et al. 2016). Study participants were recruited from two predominantly Hispanic housing projects and one local community health center. They attended weekly 90-minute sessions for 6 weeks. Based on pre- and posttest data, the culturally tailored Spanish-language cardiovascular disease prevention program showed knowledge improvements after the program (Romero et al. 2016).

Mental Health Literacy Interventions

Seventeen articles reported interventions to increase knowledge about mental health, increase confidence in identifying a person with a mental health problem, and reduce social stigma about mental illness. The majority of the mental health literacy studies focused on depression, psychosis, and stigma, though other topics were covered. Communities participating in these interventions varied by occupation (coaches, police officers, college students, farmers, community health workers, and foster care workers), age (older adults, school-aged youth), and race/ethnicity (Asian, Latino,

African American). Intervention formats included traditional class settings, workshops for adult and student groups, and use of illustrated novels (fotonovelas).

The review identified seven papers using the Mental Health First Aid (MHFA) curriculum, a standard program in community mental health literacy research (Kitchener and Jorm 2008). The intervention focuses on improving knowledge, behavior, and attitudes toward people with mental health problems and encourages help-seeking and self-help strategies. The course is typically delivered in a group setting over multiple sessions for a total of twelve hours; however, two interventions used 4-hour courses (Armstrong et al. 2011; Hart, Jorm, and Paxton 2012). Most articles describing an MHFA program included a topical breakdown of content used in training, such as an introduction to mental health disorders, mental health first aid, and practice-based skills (Armstrong et al. 2011).

Several interventions used a questionnaire to assess mental health literacy, which included vignettes about depression and schizophrenia/psychosis. The questionnaire and vignettes can be translated into community members' preferred languages and tailored in duration and delivery. Only one article described qualitative findings on use of MHFA in diverse community groups, including social workers, religious leaders, and health professionals (Svensson, Hansson, and Stjernswärd 2015). Six focus groups were held to understand how the MHFA course influenced participants. Benefits of the course were described, including understanding and humility toward people with mental illness and useful advice on handling a mental health illness crisis.

Three interventions decreased stigmatizing attitudes about mental illness (Anderson and Pierce 2012; Armstrong et al. 2011; Lam, Jorm, and Wong 2010; Wong et al. 2017). In addition to reducing stigma in adult Chinese immigrants in Melbourne, Australia, Lam and colleagues increased the participants' ability to recognize symptoms for depression and schizophrenia as well as improved beliefs about treatment, though there was no change in beliefs about seeking professional services for treatment (Lam, Jorm, and Wong et al. 2010). In another study focused on Chinese adults living in Hong Kong, Wong et al. (2017) improved participants' ability to recognize symptoms of depression and schizophrenia and confidence in offering help to others. Similar to the Lam study, Wong and colleagues (2017) did not see a decrease in perceived dangerousness and dependency and suggested that traditional Chinese beliefs about mental health may require long-term strategies to change. Anderson and Pierce (2012) trained coaches and leaders of sports teams in rural settings in Australia to improve their understanding of mental health conditions, increase their confidence in assisting those with mental illness, and decrease stigma. Results indicated an increase in knowledge regarding their reported ability to identify depression and schizophrenia/psychosis. Half of the coaches demonstrated an increase in self-confidence about helping someone experiencing mental illness, and stigma was reduced for three of every four participants. Armstrong and colleagues (2011) trained community health workers within rural communities in India to reduce stigma, but there was only evidence of a minor reduction. However, ineffective but culture-typical pharmacological interventions (vitamins, herbal medicines, and appetite stimulants) to treat mental health conditions decreased, and three months after course completion, participants' ability to identify depression and psychosis remained statistically significant.

The Mental Health First Aid curriculum has been applied to other topic areas, such as preventing eating disorders (Hart, Jorm, and Paxton 2012) and raising awareness of drought-related mental health problems (Hart, Berry, and Tonna 2011). Hart and colleagues (2012) trained college students living in residence halls at the University of Melbourne to improve knowledge, behavior, and attitudes toward people with eating disorders. Though there was no change in knowledge like other studies, participants demonstrated improved ability to recognize an eating disorder and appropriate mental health strategies, such as knowledge of effective treatments and informal help seeking. Hart, Berry, and Tonna (2011) described a program for people living in rural communities of New South Wales who had experienced severe drought. The intervention aimed to raise awareness among community members and rural farmers about mental health literacy and the effects of the drought on mental health resilience through community events. The program generated a free mental health telephone crisis line that received more than 270 calls from local farmers; booklets about local mental health services; and multiple community events and forums to raise awareness about mental health issues.

In addition to the seven MHFA studies, an additional 10 papers in this section represented a wide variety of mental health interventions. Two studies focused on reducing mental illness stigma (Fung et al. 2016; Pinto-Foltz, Logsdon, and Myers 2011). Fung and colleagues recruited adolescents and adults in Hong Kong for five interactive 3.5-hour workshops. Findings demonstrated that both adolescent and adult intervention group participants increased mental health literacy and decreased stigma. Researchers observed that education is more effective for adolescents whereas contact is more important for adults. A 10-week program, called "In Our Own Voice," used narrative storytelling and videos to reduce mental illness stigma and improve mental health literacy in a sample of 13- to 17-year-old girls attending two urban public high schools (Pinto-Foltz, Logsdon, and Myers 2011). Unlike the Fung intervention, stigma did not change post-intervention; however, mental health literacy scores increased at 4- and 8-week follow up.

Three interventions aimed to improve "dementia literacy" (Noble,

Hedmann, and Williams 2015; Rodriguez 2015; Taylor et al. 2012). Noble and colleagues used a program called Old SCHOOL (Seniors Can Have Optimal Aging and Ongoing Longevity) Hip-Hop to train fourth and fifth grade students attending a school in Harlem, New York, using three 1-hour sessions with music, role-play skits, and short films to overcome cultural barriers and beliefs about Alzheimer's and dementia, familiarize students with symptoms, and develop an appropriate response to them. Knowledge of symptoms about Alzheimer's disease increased after the intervention and was retained at the three-month follow-up. Researchers developed a 16-minute DVD titled "Looking Out for Dementia" to educate three Aboriginal communities in Australia about dementia (Taylor et al. 2012). Findings reveal increased awareness about dementia as a health issue, appreciation by communities receiving information in their native language, and the need to describe dementia as a term that does not have a comparable term in some languages. A fotonovela educational intervention designed to increase knowledge of dementia and the benefits of early diagnosis was implemented in 13 community college and adult night school classes with English- or Spanish-speaking adults (Rodriguez 2015). Compared with a brochure with dementia content and Latino family photos and a brochure with no dementia content and Latino family photos, the fotonovela content was rated most highly by participants, although both the fotonovela and brochure with dementia content and culturally appropriate photos elicited knowledge increases.

Fotonovelas were also used in two additional studies (Hernandez and Organista 2013; Unger et al. 2013). Hernandez and Organista trained promotoras to deliver fotonovelas with depression and stigma information to Latinas 18 to 55 years old and at high risk for depression. This intervention increased depression literacy, decreased stigma, and increased help-seeking knowledge and behavior. Unger and colleagues used the Secret Feelings fotonovela in a Hispanic community to increase knowledge about depression. Knowledge gain was higher in the group receiving the fotonovela compared to those who received a text pamphlet. Stigma decreased significantly in the intervention group, though scores regressed to near baseline at follow-up. Participants who received the fotonovela were more likely to report they shared the fotonovela with more than one other person compared to the group receiving the text pamphlet.

Two papers described the effect of community health workers delivering mental health literacy programs in rural villages in India (Mindlis et al. 2015; Shidhaye et al. 2017). Mindlis and colleagues assigned villages to the intervention group if they had received CHW training to support their village needs, mental health education workshops, and community reintegration activities for people with mental health conditions. Intervention villages demonstrated increased mental health literacy about depression and lower levels of stigma; however, both intervention and control villages retained a fear of medications because of potential addictive effects. Findings suggest that tailored interventions localized by village and delivered by CHWs may positively influence mental health literacy. Shidhaye and colleagues implemented a community education program (VISHRAM) in 15 rural villages in Vidarbha, India, to address mental health and suicide. CHWs conducted small group meetings and home visits, established partnerships, and obtained buy-in from key stakeholders. The result was increased demand for mental health literacy services. Requests for treatment increased six-fold over the 18-month implementation and reached more than 1,400 participants. Another important finding was a decrease in the median cost of care from baseline, which was attributed to the likelihood that villagers no longer had to seek care in the private sector, but obtained specialist services locally and at no cost, and CHWs advocated for mental health support and care.

Dowrick and colleagues (2013) aimed to increase understanding of and access to mental health services and described the "output" as improved health literacy. They designed an intervention to work at the community, health care system, and policy levels. Their target community was older adults and South Asian and Somali adults in the United Kingdom. The researchers used community engagement, primary care quality improvement, and tailored psychosocial services to provide improved service access. Group interventions were offered over 8 to 10 weeks for 1 to 2 hours each and presented case examples of people experiencing anxiety and depression. Primary care practices also received training. Qualitative evaluation suggests that participants in the intervention group who received the well-being program improved in comparison to those receiving usual care.

Two studies trained participants to assist individuals with mental illness or to counsel children (Hansson and Markström 2014; Mosuro, Malcolm, and Guishard-Pine 2014). Swedish police officers were trained over 3 weeks for a total of 31 hours on mental health literacy (Hansson and Markström 2014). The training included a video about various types of mental health conditions and the opportunity for students to role-play potential situations. The intervention group demonstrated an improved attitude toward people with mental illness, confidence in assisting someone with mental illness in accessing help, belief that medication and psychotherapy can help, and belief that people with mental illness can fully recover. Mosuro, Malcolm, and Guishard-Pine (2014) enrolled foster caregivers (parents/caretakers) in Great Britain in a nationally accredited 30-hour course modified for foster caregivers that uses didactic teaching and role-play sessions. The course was designed to increase caregivers' confidence in their mental health knowledge and ability to help counsel the children in their care. The post-course assessment demonstrated increased mental health awareness, but no impact on coping skills.

Following a devastating earthquake in Japan, Tuerk and colleagues (2013) developed an intervention to assess mental health literacy in the adult population of Mito, Japan. Participants completed questionnaires about feelings and experiences of posttraumatic stress during the 2.5-hour training. Forty-one participants turned in their questionnaires after the training. Results showed that 27 percent met criteria for posttraumatic stress disorder and 15 percent reported the earthquake was the index event. Other findings from the surveys included problems of physical health in the past 7 days and a lost sense of community. The researchers suggested that interventions such as these can address citizen concerns, inform subsequent outreach and training efforts, and help community members learn how others respond to natural disasters.

Interventions on Medicines and Health Literacy

Six articles in the review pertain to medicine and health literacy. Outcomes of interest were knowledge, self-efficacy, and communication skills.

Two studies used games to deliver an intervention. The first recruited adults ages 18 to 64 from an urban, multiethnic community setting to assess how interactive, educational board games influenced participants' knowledge about medicines and communication skills with their pharmacist (Burghardt et al. 2013). Participants who played the games were significantly more likely to report intent to seek pharmacist medication advice in the future compared to control group participants. The second study to use games was a dissertation focused on older adults living independently in a retirement community (Creech 2014). Older adults participated in a single session about medicine safety as part of a longer health class. The author used the Newest Vital Sign tool to assess health literacy (Weiss et al. 2005). Results demonstrated an increase in knowledge, but not in self-efficacy.

Adherence was the focus of two studies in this review. The first describes a school-based program in Taiwan (Chang et al. 2015). Pharmacists and teachers developed a course to help primary and middle school students communicate with their doctors, read medicine labels and instructions, assume responsibility for taking their own medicines, and talk with their pharmacists. Researchers noted an increase in knowledge, self-efficacy, and skills in the intervention groups compared with the control groups. The second study on adherence focused on older adults attending an inner city day center (Martin, Kripalani, and DuRapau 2012). Researchers instructed participants on use of a personalized, illustrated daily medicine schedule, PictureRx. Participants also completed baseline measures, including one for health literacy using the Newest Vital Sign (Weiss et al. 2005). Twenty-five percent of participants had limited health literacy, and another 25 percent had a diagnosis of dementia. Six weeks later participants were reassessed. Findings demonstrated that medicine adherence and self-efficacy improved after the intervention. Following the study, changes in program protocol included using teach-back methods by nursing staff and revising medicine instructions to avoid acronyms, using plain text descriptions instead.

Two studies focused on increasing knowledge about antibiotics and complementary and alternative therapies. David and colleagues (2017) delivered a 60-minute seminar modeled after the Ask Me 3 communication campaign to educate adults 18 and older about antibiotic resistance. Researchers used the Newest Vital Sign to assess participants recruited through local churches and YMCAs (Weiss et al. 2005). The slide presentation described the differences between viruses and bacteria, provided examples of when antibiotic use is appropriate, explained how antibiotics work, defined antibiotic resistance and examples of what could cause antibiotic resistance, and outlined steps to decrease misuse. Knowledge scores increased, but the authors noted that health literacy affected knowledge gains particularly in those with limited health literacy. Adults over age 65 living in a rural community participated in a 7-week course about complementary and alternative therapies (Shreffler-Grant, Nichols, and Weinert 2017). The course used face-to-face classes and webinars, and provided take-home materials for participants. Researchers assessed health literacy using the Newest Vital Sign (Weiss et al. 2005), the Chew Health Literacy Screener (Chew et al. 2008), and a scale specific to complementary and alternative therapy literacy. Findings demonstrated that health literacy mean scores increased, but were not statistically significant.

Cancer and Health Literacy

Eight papers reported health literacy interventions about cancer focused primarily on increasing knowledge and self-efficacy. Most of the studies focused on women, and three of the studies addressed cost.

Culturally tailored and peer-led interventions were used to increase knowledge about breast and cervical cancer. Using promotoras to facilitate the six-week course, *Nuestra Cocina: Mesa Buena, Vida Sana*, researchers delivered a cooking class to Latinas over age 40 (Castañeda et al. 2016). Topics in the course addressed women's health and cancer basics, navigation of screening services, myths about breast cancer, communication with providers, and risk reduction strategies. Findings demonstrated an increase in knowledge and a greater likelihood of having a mammogram or colorectal cancer exam after the intervention. However, there was no significant increase in health literacy as measured by the Chew Health Literacy Screener, which assessed for confidence in filling out medical forms, asking for help reading medical material, and interpreting written medications (Chew et al. 2008). Korean-American women from 23 ethnic churches in an urban setting participated in an intervention about breast and cervical cancer screening. Community health workers received training and later trained participants in CHW homes, food courts, and ethnic cafes and grocery stores (Han et al. 2017). Workshops were designed to build health literacy skills regarding medical terminology about screening, medical instructions, and steps to navigate the health care system. Following the intervention, CHWs conducted monthly phone calls with participants and provided navigation support for up to six months. The researchers used an Assessment of Health Literacy in Cancer Screening (52 items), which assesses print literacy, numeracy, and cancer-specific terms. The intervention group had a higher likelihood of receiving mammograms and cervical cancer screening at a 6-month follow-up compared with control participants. Researchers assessed cost-effectiveness using an incremental cost effectiveness ratio. The cost per screening for someone in the intervention group to receive screening compared with someone in the comparison group was $236. More details about the cost-effectiveness study can be obtained in Schuster et al. (2015).

Two studies designed interventions on empowerment for adolescents and young adults. Researchers used a cervical cancer education program called the "Sexual Health Empowerment (SHE) Project" delivered to women over age 18 in a county jail in Kansas City, Kansas (Ramaswamy, Simmons, and Kelly 2015). Session topics focused on increasing knowledge, reducing perceived barriers, improving self-efficacy and ability to communicate with providers, and navigating the health care system. Results demonstrated increased scores in knowledge about cervical cancer, increased self-efficacy for screening, and increased confidence in navigating providers and health systems. In a qualitative evaluation of the After Cancer Care Ends, Survivorship Starts for Adolescent and Young Adults (ACCESS AYA), researchers explored how it improved health literacy among participants. The participants included community health providers, AYA survivors, caregivers, and cancer advocates. One important finding among AYA survivors was the desire to practice self and community advocacy, which may be tied to the program's emphasis on self-advocacy with medical professionals. AYA survivors also described increased knowledge and establishing community connections with other survivors. Cancer advocates reinforced the need for education and dissemination of materials as well as in-person group meetings for survivors to share information and experiences.

Environmental Health Risks, Communication, and Behaviors

Two papers reported interventions to clearly communicate environmental data and information in communities affected by health hazards (Paul et al. 2015; Ramirez-Andreotta et al. 2016). Both sets of researchers noted that communicating environmental risk data and recommendations in ways that motivate health-protective behaviors is especially challenging. One article used health literacy as the core concept (Paul et al. 2015), and the other used environmental health literacy, which they define as an "understanding of the connection between environmental exposures and human health" (Ramirez-Andreotta et al. 2016). A paper on well water contamination identified low health literacy in the community as a contributing factor to low levels of recommended water-testing behaviors (Paul et al. 2015). Community presentations on health risks and protective actions, an information campaign, community distribution of water kits, and test results produced a three-fold increase in water testing. In the other intervention, researchers did two home visits with residents living in a Superfund designated area (Ramirez-Andreotta et al. 2016). Researchers took biological samples from residents and environmental samples around the home. They also collected resident information with a questionnaire and asked residents to complete activity duration and dietary logs for the 4 days before the second home visit. Residents received individual and summary toxicity-level reports and phone calls to discuss results. The community hosted three meetings. An evaluation showed residents used the information to cope, change family household behaviors, and take steps to reduce exposures.

Policy/System Intervention

The review identified one paper reporting the effects of a national health policy change in Sweden that the authors stated was intended to increase population health literacy skills (Mahmud et al. 2010). The policy emphasized primary care, more individual responsibility for self-care, and population health. County councils were expected to provide local primary care services (health squares) and health promotion initiatives to strengthen health and health literacy in communities. Researchers were interested in how the policy was implemented at local levels and how well it supported the policy goals. They analyzed thirty "health squares" (primary care centers) and found that people's limited understanding of health promotion and empowerment concepts was a weakness, but a strength was a wide choice of health information materials and individualized counseling with staff. The authors suggest that the actors in the policy/community process should build a common understanding of health promotion and empowerment so the policy could be implemented as intended.

Excluded Papers of Interest for Community Health Literacy Interventions

Some excluded papers described interventions with interesting features relevant for community-based health literacy interventions. Although the interventions did not match the inclusion criteria, the team believes the papers can foster discussion about how health literacy insights can contribute to the broad domain of community-based interventions. Some excluded papers may also suggest potential research partnerships and intervention designs that can benefit from health literacy insights.

Authors of included papers discussed their challenges in recruiting large numbers of community members or entire communities to participate in research. Therefore, three excluded papers on health literacy issues for recruitment and retention of community members in research studies are of special interest (Nagler et al. 2013; Pelto et al. 2016; Rexroth and Friedland 2010). These papers were not included in the review because they did not describe interventions and outcomes, but they could inform dialogues on community engagement and "research adherence," that is, a community's sustained interest and participation in research. Community members' interest, willingness, and continued participation in a study could be a valuable community intervention outcome with health literacy being a prime contributor.

Three interventions helped health profession students be more effective communicators by interacting with community-dwelling members outside health care visits (Grice et al. 2014; Hjertstedt, Barnes, and Sjostedt 2014; Milford et al. 2016). These papers were excluded because the interventions focused on educating the students to interact one-on-one with individual community residents. Nevertheless, these interventions showed opportunities to get health professionals "out of the classroom and into the community," as the title of one paper put it (Milford et al. 2016). One intervention trained first and second year medical students to counsel Head Start children, parents, and staff on pediatric obesity prevention (Milford et al. 2016). An intervention for dental students sent them into older adults' homes to educate them about oral health and measure their oral health literacy and oral health status (Hjertstedt, Barnes, and Sjostedt 2014). Third-year pharmacy students were assigned to older adults living in senior housing (Grice et al. 2014). The students used health literacy techniques such as Ask Me 3 and teach-back to collect health histories, do safety checks, and assess medicine use, among other tasks.

One study used an interesting environmental intervention design to increase health literacy, but was excluded because people were recruited as individuals (Crim 2013). University faculty and staff were the target of an intervention to affect individually perceived health literacy and purchasing behaviors in on-campus eateries. The researcher designed and implemented a red, yellow, and green point-of-purchase labeling system to rate foods. Color-coded stickers, lighted menu boards, posters, emails, and table tents communicated the rating system. Exposure times were varied across the eateries: one eatery had the intervention for 6 weeks, the second for 4 weeks, and the third for 2 weeks. Comparing responses from a paper-and-pencil pretest and an online survey posttest, 42 percent of respondents said the color coding influenced their awareness, understanding, and food choices, but not intentions or knowledge. There was a significant increase in "green" food sales and a significant decrease in "red" food sales, regardless of length of intervention.

Two examples—one from Bangladesh and the other from Venezuela—hint at how community-level interventions could be designed with health literacy outcomes that extend beyond individual knowledge and behavior change. Since the mid-1990s, a research group in Bangladesh has helped build communities' capacity to address their own problems (Bhuiya, Hanifi, and Hoque 2016). Using a Participatory Rural Appraisal model, the researchers worked with rural, village-run organizations on a "self-help for health" program. The stated purpose was to build organizational capacity to address collective health problems, improve health literacy through individual awareness related to health improvements, and support participatory planning and monitoring in villages. Using intervention and comparison communities, surveys, project documents and workplans, and reports, researchers reported a number of improvements in the intervention community, including more organizational capacity as well as better health outcomes, such as lower infant mortality and increased vaccination. However, health literacy was mentioned only in the abstract, and villagers' literacy rates were mentioned only in passing in the body of the paper. The paper does not explain what the intervention did to improve literacy or health literacy and if there were any changes.

In a second example, researchers in Venezuela described an advocacy and social mobilization intervention over a 4-year period to increase health literacy about breast cancer in Venezuela (Eid and Nahon-Serfaty 2015). They used health literacy as the justification as well as the proposed outcome, but did not explain how the campaign incorporated or tried to affect health literacy. Nongovernmental organizations, physicians, scholars, journalists, public officials from state and municipal governments, and women who had experienced breast cancer created an action-oriented network to develop advocates and activists, enhance patient–provider communication, and promote social dialogue among stakeholders. The network organized multiple activities such as national campaigns, a cancer walk, educational materials, digital media, conferences, and public opinion forums. Annual workshops taught attendees how to create messages about breast health to promote attitudinal and behavioral changes. The focus of these efforts culminated in mobilizing multiple levels of local communities and national organizations for a national policy on breast cancer. However, the researchers did not report specific health literacy components.

DISCUSSION

This review's results show the existence of a wide variety of community-based health literacy interventions. These interventions have positively affected several types of outcomes for many different groups of people. The outcomes range from knowledge gain to changes in social norms, health care service use, or physiological measures, with knowledge change being the most frequent outcome. As noted in the results section, however, relatively few papers reported quantifiable results expressed as pre- and posttest differences between intervention and comparison groups. Many studies were designed with only an intervention group measured with pre- and posttests, leading to a finding that was not especially surprising—that knowledge usually increased, as did related outcomes such as self-efficacy. In addition to these results, four broad themes emerged from the full-text review.

Community Engagement in Planning and Implementing Interventions

The first theme pertains to the seriousness with which researchers are engaging with communities to design interventions. The many positive results may reflect, in part, that interventions frequently incorporated community perspectives and input even at formative stages, leading to interventions that participants often characterized as a good fit. High levels of community involvement at multiple stages in the intervention process are appropriate and admirable for health literacy improvement work. To the degree that health literacy and cultural competence are conceptually linked, community involvement ensures that interventions are relevant, understandable, and useful in helping communities to protect and promote health. Also, community specificity may partially account for the number of unique intervention designs and implementations, a low number of randomized trials, and frequent use of qualitative evaluations and self-report data in the final set of papers.

A few papers illustrated intervention failure when community perspectives were not appropriately considered. An evaluation found that school-based health programs for immigrant and culturally marginal school children and parents in Spain often ignored the *expressed needs of the community* and community members' *cultural intelligence* (italics in original)

(Flecha, García, and Rudd 2011). The researchers concluded "the course [on how to keep children from being involved with drugs] failed because the abilities and knowledge that the participants had acquired from their experience with drugs in their families were ignored" (Flecha, García, and Rudd 2011, 213). The negative consequences for health literacy were that family members did not have sufficient trust in the school and teachers as information sources and were less interested in participating in the planned activities.

Community specificity may also help account for the low number of replicated interventions, with the Mental Health First Aid and Ophelia models being notable exceptions. The Australian adult literacy program and the U.S. Meals on Wheels health coaches adapted existing interventions for new communities (Beauchamp et al. 2017; Muscat et al. 2016; Rubin et al. 2014). Researchers were more likely to create their own materials and programs, and sometimes measurement tools, than to try an intervention effective with a different community, setting, or topic. Encouraging researchers to publicly share their instruments, materials, and program designs may motivate more adaptation or replication with appropriate cultural considerations. A few research teams have posted their materials online: Georgia Meals on Wheels (Rubin et al. 2014), the Australian Ophelia model (Beauchamp et al. 2017), and *Buenos Hábitos Alimenticios para una Buena Salud* (Otilingam et al. 2015).

Reporting back to communities characterizes community-engaged research, although report-back is not an element in the CDC Best Practices framework nor an activity the included papers typically addressed. Two excluded papers did not report interventions, but did discuss the health literacy and ethical issues as well as experiences and recommended practices for reporting biomonitoring and environmental exposures to individuals and communities (Brody et al. 2014; Ohayon et al. 2017). The papers indicate that reporting back clear and useful information to communities should be the norm. One set of authors concludes, "Thoughtful report-back can strengthen research experiences for investigators and participants and expand the translation of environmental health research in communities" (Brody et al. 2014, 40).

Health Literacy Components of Interventions

A second theme pertains to the way "health literacy" was used in interventions. The review team did not have preconceived ideas about when and how health literacy would appear in an intervention. Instead, through the review process, four ways emerged regarding how health literacy was included at one or more points in an intervention. The papers included described interventions that (a) identified or characterized the community of interest as "low health literate"; (b) used a health literacy instrument or measure to advance the analysis; (c) designed programs or materials using health literacy principles or techniques; or (d) assessed changes in knowledge, self-efficacy, skills, behaviors, or other outcomes that authors considered to be included in health literacy or related to health literacy. Table C-8 refers to these possible loci of health literacy in interventions as (a) community, (b) measurement, (c) content, or (d) outcome, respectively. On the one hand, the appearance of health literacy considerations at multiple points in an intervention is a positive sign that researchers take health literacy seriously as a pervasive factor in intervention effectiveness. On the other hand, the lack of consistency in using these four elements (or others the field may be interested in) is a sign that researchers do not share a common view of when health literacy should be considered in interventions.

Some examples illustrate problems created when the health literacy concept is inconsistently applied. During the full-text review, the review team excluded many articles that used "health literacy" in the title or abstract only and not in the body of the paper. The interventions were typically trying to increase knowledge and sometimes self-efficacy, empowerment, or other factors related to health attitudes and behaviors; and to change one or more health behaviors. The papers, however, did not address explicitly the four health literacy components. In a school-based health program to change family knowledge and behaviors for diabetes, researchers aimed to train healthy adolescents to become health coaches for family members with diabetes (Gefter et al. 2016). The researchers described a group—low-income ethnic minority students from families with diabetes—with a high likelihood of having low health literacy. However, the researchers do not report health literacy measures, techniques, or outcomes for the students or intervention; yet, the abstract conclusion says "this program can increase health knowledge and some psychosocial assets of at-risk youth and holds promise to empower these youth with *health literacy* [emphasis added] and encourage them to adopt healthy behaviors" (Gefter et al. 2016). A culturally adapted cardiovascular risk reduction program for African Americans manifests a similar approach (Brewer et al. 2016). The researchers describe many contextual factors that would suggest limited health literacy being a major consideration for both community members and the intervention implementation and results. However, health literacy was not evident in the intervention itself or the actual results.

At the very least, inconsistencies in the ways "health literacy" is invoked in an intervention can create problems when developing coherent reporting schemes for comparative reviews such as this one. From a scientific perspective, the lack of explicit and consistent use of "health literacy" to inform intervention design, implementation, and reporting may impede building the body of knowledge about what characterizes effective and ineffective community-based health literacy interventions. As evidenced by the examples above, interventions may also append "health literacy" without sufficient evidence to warrant the connection.

Health Literacy and Knowledge Outcomes

The review team expected to find many knowledge-building interventions, and the third discussion theme pertains to how to think about knowledge improvement as a community intervention outcome. Although increasing health knowledge is popular, it can also be a disparaged outcome when researchers, practitioners, and policy makers expect every intervention to result in a behavior or health status change. The review team found many community interventions aimed to increase participants' knowledge of a health topic or general health care. Because it is axiomatic that educational interventions nearly always increase short- if not medium-term knowledge, it would be easy to dismiss knowledge interventions and results as finding the obvious. From another perspective, however, the large number of knowledge-building interventions is also a sign of a fundamental and structural problem in many communities. In addition to the well-documented problem that many health information materials are a poor match for people's skills, the studies in this review also show large-scale problems with communities' limited information awareness and access. Even in countries such as the United States that have universal public education and an abundance of communication channels and information sources, low levels of health knowledge are an ongoing problem; moreover, prior research shows health knowledge and health literacy are related (Dennison et al. 2011; Hom et al. 2012; Williams et al. 1998). The studies included paint a picture of many communities cut off from the large amount and variety of health information that exists beyond their personal and collective experiences. As a team of Australian researchers observed about the adult education students in their intervention, "Students had limited or no formal experience learning about issues regarding their health" (Muscat et al. 2016, 5).

One excluded paper, a cardiac risk reduction intervention with African-American church-goers in Rochester, Minnesota (Brewer et al. 2016), provides information about the large and ongoing need to build knowledge in communities, as well as the limited role that health literacy insights have played in shaping many community interventions. The researchers for this intervention note an abundance of information about how to prevent cardiovascular disease and examples of successful cardiac risk reduction interventions for African Americans, and yet there is an extremely low level of ideal cardiac health among African Americans. But this information had not diffused in the African American community in Rochester. The intervention came about when three African American churches in Rochester asked local researchers for help with a health and wellness program. The researchers introduced church-goers to a culturally adapted version of *Life's Simple 7*, the American Heart Association's cardiac risk reduction program. Not surprisingly, researchers found they had to tackle low levels of cardiac health knowledge as well as other factors to show improvements in health outcomes. This study and many others in the review suggest that low levels of knowledge about reliable health information remain an ongoing problem that could negatively affect the development of higher level skills, such as effective communication and critical analysis. A continued focus on knowledge building as part of health literacy interventions may be necessary because communities often come to interventions isolated from the larger universe of science-based health information and lacking foundational knowledge that affects health literacy.

Challenges Applying an Evaluation Framework

The last discussion theme addresses the fit between evaluation frameworks for generally-used public health interventions and the community-based health literacy interventions in this review. The review team considered several evaluation models before selecting the CDC Best Practices framework (Spencer et al. 2013). The framework assesses the impact and quality of real-world programs to improve health and includes the general categories of Effectiveness, Reach, Feasibility, Sustainability, and Transferability. Each general category has several subcomponents. The framework includes a separate set of criteria about evidence quality, but the review team did not agree with definitions for "weak," "moderate," and "strong" evidence. The team specifically disagreed with the rating that all peer-reviewed studies are "strong" in quality. The team decided not to use the Best Practices evidence quality categories and instead reported on the study design categories from the *Guide to Community Preventive Services* (HHS 2001).

The review team applied the CDC Best Practices framework to individual papers, but the framework was not especially useful for identifying papers for inclusion. Few papers had the majority of the information in the framework, especially under Feasibility, Sustainability, and Transferability. The team included as much information about Effectiveness and Reach as papers reported. However, under the Effectiveness category, the majority of papers did not report the magnitude of the effects; the significance of the intervention and results; the benefits or risks of the intervention for the intended population/group; or how the intervention contributed to health equity. Under the Reach category, papers typically did not discuss how many people the researchers intended to reach or could have reached with the intervention. The review template is included as Tables C-5, C-6, and

C-7 in the hope that it will stimulate discussion about future intervention design and reporting. For the current review, the Best Practices framework categories appear better suited to be guides to what community health literacy interventions should consider and report than helpful pointers to evaluate what has already been published.

CONCLUSION

The Horowitz Center review team identified a wide variety of community-based health literacy interventions, encompassing different communities, topics, settings, and outcomes. Researchers applied the health literacy concept to choose communities of interest; design or apply measures; design or adapt materials and programs; and identify outcomes. Although few included papers reported the magnitude of effects, they did contain a wide range of qualitative and quantitative data that can be used to inform future research; knowledge change was the most frequent outcome. Many of the challenges in conducting the review came from distinguishing between health literacy and health education interventions and between individual and community-based interventions. The team also grappled with the frequent ambiguities in the role health literacy played in defining relevant outcomes. The final included set of papers reflects the team's assessment that however difficult it is to draw meaningful distinctions, they can be drawn, and the tensions produced by the exercise can be interesting and productive in advancing health literacy and public health theory and practice.

REFERENCES

Anderson, R. J., and D. Pierce. 2012. "Assumptions Associated with Mental Health Literacy Training: Insights from Initiatives in Rural Australia." *Advances in Mental Health* 10(3):258–267. doi: 10.5172/jamh.2012.10.3.258.

APA (American Psychological Association). 2010. *Publication Manual of the American Psychological Association*. 6th ed. Washington, DC: APA.

Arksey, H., and L. O'Malley. 2005. "Scoping Studies: Towards a Methodological Framework." *International Journal of Social Research Methodology* 8(1):19–32. doi: 10.1080/1364557032000119616.

Armstrong, G., M. Kermode, S. Raja, S. Suja, P. Chandra, and A. F. Jorm. 2011. "A Mental Health Training Program for Community Health Workers in India: Impact on Knowledge and Attitudes." *International Journal of Mental Health Systems* 5:17. doi: 10.1186/1752-4458-5-17.

Ayub, R. A., T. Jaffery, F. Aziz, and M. Rahmat. 2015. "Improving Health Literacy of Women about Iron Deficiency Anemia and Civic Responsibility of Students through Service Learning." *Education for Health* 28(2):130. doi: 10.4103/1357-6283.170122.

Batterham, R. W., R. Buchbinder, A. Beauchamp, S. Dodson, G. R. Elsworth, and R. H. Osborne. 2014. "The OPtimising HEalth LIterAcy (OPHELIA) Process: Study Protocol for Using Health Literacy Profiling and Community Engagement to Create and Implement Health Reform." *BMC Public Health* 14(July):694. doi: 10.1186/1471-2458-14-694.

Beauchamp, A., R. W. Batterham, S. Dodson, B. Astbury, G. R. Elsworth, C. McPhee, J. Jacobson, R. Buchbinder, and R. H. Osborne. 2017. "Systematic Development and Implementation of Interventions to OPtimise Health Literacy and Access (Ophelia)." *BMC Public Health* 17:230. doi: 10.1186/s12889-017-4147-5.

Berkman, N. D., S. L. Sheridan, K. E. Donahue, D. J. Halpern, A. Viera, K. Crotty, A. Holland et al. 2011. "Health Literacy Interventions and Outcomes: An Updated Systematic Review." *Evidence Report/Technology Assessment* 199(March):1–941.

Bertera, E. M. 2014. "Storytelling Slide Shows to Improve Diabetes and High Blood Pressure Knowledge and Self-Efficacy: Three-Year Results Among Community Dwelling Older African Americans." *Educational Gerontology* 40(11):785–800. doi: 10.1080/03601277.2014.894381.

Bhuiya, A., S. M. A. Hanifi, and S. Hoque. 2016. "Unlocking Community Capability through Promotion of Self-Help for Health: Experience from Chakaria, Bangladesh." *BMC Health Services Research* 16(7):624. doi: 10.1186/s12913-016-1865-9.

Brewer, L. C., J. E. Balls-Berry, P. Dean, K. Lackore, S. Jenkins, and S. N. Hayes. 2016. "Fostering African-American Improvement in Total Health (FAITH!): An Application of the American Heart Association's Life's Simple 7™ among Midwestern African-Americans." *Journal of Racial and Ethnic Health Disparities* 4(2):269–281. doi: 10.1007/s40615-016-0226-z.

Brody, J. G., S. C. Dunagan, R. Morello-Frosch, P. Brown, S. Patton, and R. A. Rudel. 2014. "Reporting Individual Results for Biomonitoring and Environmental Exposures: Lessons Learned from Environmental Communication Case Studies." *Environmental Health: A Global Access Science Source* 13(May):40. doi: 10.1186/1476-069X-13-40.

Brown, N., V. Collie-Akers, and C. Fernandez-Ortega. 2015. "Merging Adult Education with Nutrition Literacy to Empower Mexican Women." In *Literacy as Gendered Discourse: Engaging the Voices of Women in Global Societies*, edited by D. W. Ntiri, pp. 133–151. Adult Education Special Topics: Theory, Research, and Practice in Lifelong Learning. Charlotte, NC: IAP.

Burgette, J. M. 2016. "The Impact of Early Head Start on Children's Oral Health." Ph.D. dissertation, Chapel Hill, NC: University of North Carolina at Chapel Hill.

Burghardt, K. J., M. R. Bowman, M. Hibino, B. K. Opong-Owusu, Jr., T. D. Pokora, K. Reeves, and K. M. Vile. 2013. "Using Educational Games to Promote the Seeking of a Pharmacist and to Teach Key Medication Use Messages: Results from an Inner City Health Party." *Research in Social and Administrative Pharmacy* 9(5):542–552. doi: 10.1016/j.sapharm.2013.01.001.

Castañeda, S. F., R. E. Giacinto, E. A. Medeiros, I. Brongiel, O. Cardona, P. Perez, and G. A. Talavera. 2016. "Academic–Community Partnership to Develop a Patient-Centered Breast Cancer Risk Reduction Program for Latina Primary Care Patients." *Journal of Racial and Ethnic Health Disparities* 3(2):189–199. doi: 10.1007/s40615-015-0125-8.

Chan, L. S. 2012. "Chronic Disease Self-Management in Hong Kong Chinese Older Adults Living in the Community." Ph.D. dissertation, Hong Kong: Chinese University of Hong Kong.

Chang, F. C., H. Y. Chi, L. J. Huang, C. H. Lee, J. L. Yang, and M. K. Yeh. 2015. "Developing School–Pharmacist Partnerships to Enhance Correct Medication Use and Pain Medication Literacy in Taiwan." *Journal of the American Pharmacists Association* 55(6):595. doi: 10.1331/JAPhA.2015.15053.

Chen, H., P. Cohen, and S. Chen. 2010. "How Big Is a Big Odds Ratio? Interpreting the Magnitudes of Odds Ratios in Epidemiological Studies." *Communications in Statistics—Simulation and Computation* 39(4):860–864. doi: 10.1080/03610911003650383.

Chervin, C., J. Clift, L. Woods, E. Krause, and K. Lee. 2012. "Health Literacy in Adult Education: A Natural Partnership for Health Equity." *Health Promotion Practice* 13(6):738–746. doi: 10.1177/1524839912437367.

Chew, L. D., J. M. Griffin, M. R. Partin, S. Noorbaloochi, J. P. Grill, A. Snyder, K. A. Bradley, S. M. Nugent, A. D. Baines, and M. VanRyn. 2008. "Validation of Screening Questions for Limited Health Literacy in a Large VA Outpatient Population." *Journal of General Internal Medicine* 23(5):561–566. doi: 10.1007/s11606-008-0520-5.

Cohen, J. 1988. *Statistical Power Analysis for the Behavioral Sciences*. 2nd ed. Hillsdale, NJ: Lawrence Erlbaum Associates.

Creech, C. L. 2014. "The 'Medication Matters ... To You!' Educational Intervention Session: A Pilot Study to Improve Medication Management in Community-Living Older Adults." Ph.D. dissertation, Denton, TX: Texas Woman's University.

Crim, B. N. 2013. "An Evaluation of a Point of Purchase Labeling Intervention to Improve Health Literacy and Healthy Eating Choices." Thesis. https://repositories.lib.utexas.edu/handle/2152/28722 (accessed June 1, 2017).

David, C. M., K. S. O'Neal, M. J. Miller, J. L. Johnson, and A. E. Lloyd. 2017. "A Literacy-Sensitive Approach to Improving Antibiotic Understanding in a Community-Based Setting." *International Journal of Pharmacy Practice*. doi: 10.1111/ijpp.12332.

Dennison, C. R., M. L. McEntee, L. Samuel, B. J. Johnson, S. Rotman, A. Kielty, and S. D. Russell. 2011. "Adequate Health Literacy Is Associated with Higher Heart Failure Knowledge and Self Care Confidence in Hospitalized Patients." *Journal of Cardiovascular Nursing* 26(5):359–367. doi: 10.1097/JCN.0b013e3181f16f88.

Diamond, C., S. Saintonge, P. August, and A. Azrack. 2011. "The Development of Building Wellness™, a Youth Health Literacy Program." *Journal of Health Communication* 16(Supplement 3):103–118. doi: 10.1080/10810730.2011.604385.

Dowrick, C., C. Chew-Graham, K. Lovell, J. Lamb, S. Aseem, S. Beatty, P. Bowe, H. Burroughs, P. Clarke, S. Edwards, M. Gabbay, K. Gravenhorst, J. Hammond, D. Hibbert, M. Kovandžić, M. Lloyd-Williams, W. Waheed, and L. Gask. 2013. *Increasing Equity of Access to High-Quality Mental Health Services in Primary Care: A Mixed-Methods Study*. Programme Grants for Applied Research. Southampton, UK: NIHR Journals Library. http://www.ncbi.nlm.nih.gov/books/NBK374112 (accessed June 1, 2017).

Eid, M., and I. Nahon-Serfaty. 2015. "Risk, Activism, and Empowerment: Women's Breast Cancer in Venezuela." *International Journal of Civic Engagement and Social Change* 2(1):43–64. doi: 10.4018/IJCESC.2015010104.

Elsworth, G. R., A. Beauchamp, and R. H. Osborne. 2016. "Measuring Health Literacy in Community Agencies: A Bayesian Study of the Factor Structure and Measurement Invariance of the Health Literacy Questionnaire (HLQ)." *BMC Health Services Research* 16(1):508. doi: 10.1186/s12913-016-1754-2.

Fleary, S. A. 2012. "A Parent-Focused Intervention to Increase Parent Health Literacy and Healthy Lifestyle Choices for Young Children and Families." Ph.D. dissertation, College Station, TX: Texas A&M University.

Flecha, A., R. García, and R. Rudd. 2011. "Using Health Literacy in School to Overcome Inequalities." *European Journal of Education* 46(2):209–218. doi: 10.1111/j.1465-3435.2011.01476.x.

Freedman, A. M. 2011. "Adult Education as a Vehicle for Health Communication." Ph.D. dissertation, Atlanta, GA: Emory University.

Fung, E., T. L. Lo, R. W. S. Chan, F. C. C. Woo, C. W. L. Ma, and B. S. M. Mak. 2016. "Outcome of a Knowledge Contact-Based Anti-Stigma Programme in Adolescents and Adults in the Chinese Population." *East Asian Archives of Psychiatry* 26(4):129–136.

Gefter, L., N. Morioka-Douglas, A. Srivastava, and E. Rodriguez. 2016. "Supporting At-Risk Youth and Their Families to Manage and Prevent Diabetes: Developing a National Partnership of Medical Residency Programs and High Schools." *PLoS ONE* 11(7):e0158477. doi: 10.1371/journal.pone.0158477.

Goeman, D., S. Conway, R. Norman, J. Morley, R. Weerasuriya, R. H. Osborne, and A. Beauchamp. 2016. "Optimising Health Literacy and Access of Service Provision to Community Dwelling Older People with Diabetes Receiving Home Nursing Support." *Journal of Diabetes Research* 2016(September):e2483263. doi: 10.1155/2016/2483263.

Goodman, M. S., J. J. Dias, and J. D. Stafford. 2010. "Increasing Research Literacy in Minority Communities: CARES Fellows Training Program." *Journal of Empirical Research on Human Research Ethics* 5(4):33–41. doi: 10.1525/jer.2010.5.4.33.

Gray, K., K. Elliott, and J. Wale. 2013. "A Community Education Initiative to Improve Using Online Health Information: Participation and Impact." *Informatics for Health & Social Care* 38(3):171–181. doi: 10.3109/17538157.2012.705201.

Grice, G. R., A. Tiemeier, P. Hurd, T. M. Berry, M. Voorhees, T. R. Prosser, J. Sailors, N. M. Gattas, and W. Duncan. 2014. "Student Use of Health Literacy Tools to Improve Patient Understanding and Medication Adherence." *The Consultant Pharmacist* 29(4): 240–253.

Han, H. R., Y. Song, M. Kim, H. K. Hedlin, K. Kim, H. Ben Lee, and D. Roter. 2017. "Breast and Cervical Cancer Screening Literacy Among Korean American Women: A Community Health Worker-Led Intervention." *American Journal of Public Health* 107(1):159–165. doi: 10.2105/AJPH.2016.303522.

Hansson, L., and U. Markström. 2014. "The Effectiveness of an Anti-Stigma Intervention in a Basic Police Officer Training Programme: A Controlled Study." *BMC Psychiatry* 14:55. doi: 10.1186/1471-244X-14-55.

Harrison, L., D. Ollis, and G. Savige. 2016. "'The Doctor Just Talks about It': Sustainable Health Promotion and Practice in Schools." August. http://dro.deakin.edu.au/view/DU:30085935 (accessed June 1, 2017).

Hart, C. R., H. L. Berry, and A. M. Tonna. 2011. "Improving the Mental Health of Rural New South Wales Communities Facing Drought and Other Adversities." *Australian Journal of Rural Health* 19(5):231–238. doi: 10.1111/j.1440-1584.2011.01225.x.

Hart, L. M., A. F. Jorm, and S. J. Paxton. 2012. "Mental Health First Aid for Eating Disorders: Pilot Evaluation of a Training Program for the Public." *BMC Psychiatry* 12:98. doi: 10.1186/1471-244X-12-98.

Hatamleh, J. 2015. "Health Literacy of Iraqi Immigrant Adults Pilot Study." Ph.D. dissertation, Akron, OH: University of Akron. http://rave.ohiolink.edu/etdc/view?acc_num=akron1447357948 (accessed June 1, 2017).

Healthy People 2020. n.d. "Health Communication and Health Information Technology." https://www.healthypeople.gov/2020/topics-objectives/topic/health-communication-and-health-information-technology (accessed June 1, 2017).

Hernandez, M. Y., and K. C. Organista. 2013. "Entertainment–Education? A Fotonovela? A New Strategy to Improve Depression Literacy and Help-Seeking Behaviors in At-Risk Immigrant Latinas." *American Journal of Community Psychology* 52(3–4):224–235. doi: 10.1007/s10464-013-9587-1.

HHS (U.S. Department of Health and Human Services). 2001. *Task Force on Community Preventive Services*. https://www.thecommunityguide.org (accessed June 1, 2017).

HHS. 2010. *National Action Plan to Improve Health Literacy*. Washington, DC: Office of Disease Prevention and Health Promotion. https://health.gov/communication/initiatives/health-literacy-action-plan.asp (accessed June 1, 2017).

Hjertstedt, J., S. L. Barnes, and J. M. Sjostedt. 2014. "Investigating the Impact of a Community-Based Geriatric Dentistry Rotation on Oral Health Literacy and Oral Hygiene of Older Adults." *Gerodontology* 31(4):296–307. doi: 10.1111/ger.12038.

Hom, J. M., J. Y. Lee, K. Divaris, A. D. Baker, and W. F. Vann. 2012. "Oral Health Literacy and Knowledge among Patients Who Are Pregnant for the First Time." *Journal of the American Dental Association* 143(9):972–980.

IOM (Institute of Medicine). 2004. *Health Literacy: A Prescription to End Confusion.* Washington, DC: The National Academies Press.

Kim, K. B., H. R. Han, B. Huh, T. Nguyen, H. Lee, and M. T. Kim. 2014. "The Effect of a Community-Based Self-Help Multimodal Behavioral Intervention in Korean American Seniors with High Blood Pressure." *American Journal of Hypertension* 27(9):1199–1208. doi: 10.1093/ajh/hpu041.

Kim, M. T., K. B. Kim, B. Huh, T. Nguyen, H. R. Han, L. R. Bone, and D. Levine. 2015. "The Effect of a Community-Based Self-Help Intervention: Korean Americans with Type 2 Diabetes." *American Journal of Preventive Medicine* 49(5):726–737. doi: 10.1016/j.amepre.2015.04.033.

Kitchener, B. A., and A. F. Jorm. 2008. "Mental Health First Aid: An International Programme for Early Intervention." *Early Intervention in Psychiatry* 2(1):55–61. doi: 10.1111/j.1751-7893.2007.00056.x.

Lam, A. Y. K., A. F. Jorm, and D. F. K. Wong. 2010. "Mental Health First Aid Training for the Chinese Community in Melbourne, Australia: Effects on Knowledge About and Attitudes Toward People with Mental Illness." *International Journal of Mental Health Systems* 4:18. doi: 10.1186/1752-4458-4-18.

Lam, H. S. 2014. "The Effect of a Health Literacy Oriented Program on Physical Activity among Chinese Patients with Type 2 Diabetes Mellitus." University of Hong Kong Libraries, University of Hong Kong. doi: 10.5353/th_b5334852.

Levin-Zamir, D., S. Keret, O. Yaakovson, B. Lev, C. Kay, G. Verber, and N. Lieberman. 2011. "Refuah Shlema: A Cross-Cultural Programme for Promoting Communication and Health among Ethiopian Immigrants in the Primary Health Care Setting in Israel: Evidence and Lessons Learned from over a Decade of Implementation." *Global Health Promotion* 18(1):51–54. doi: 10.1177/1757975910393172.

Mahmud, A. J., E. Olander, L. Wallenberg, and B. J. A. Haglund. 2010. "Health Promoting Settings in Primary Health Care—'Hälsotorg': An Implementation Analysis." *BMC Public Health* 10:707. doi: 10.1186/1471-2458-10-707.

Mancuso, L. 2011. "Overcoming Health Literacy Barriers: A Model for Action." *Journal of Cultural Diversity; Lisle* 18(2):60–65.

Martin, D., S. Kripalani, and V. J. DuRapau. 2012. "Improving Medication Management Among At-Risk Older Adults." *Journal of Gerontological Nursing; Thorofare* 38(6):24–34. doi:http://dx.doi.org/10.3928/00989134-20120507-50.

McLeroy, K. R., B. L. Norton, M. C. Kegler, J. N. Burdine, and C. V. Sumaya. 2003. "Community-Based Interventions." *American Journal of Public Health* 93(4):529–533. doi: 10.2105/AJPH.93.4.529.

Milford, E., K. Morrison, C. Teutsch, B. B. Nelson, A. Herman, M. King, and N. Beucke. 2016. "Out of the Classroom and Into the Community: Medical Students Consolidate Learning About Health Literacy Through Collaboration with Head Start." *BMC Medical Education* 16:121. doi: 10.1186/s12909-016-0635-z.

Mindlis, I., J. Schuetz-Mueller, S. Shah, R. Appasani, A. Coleman, and C. L. Katz. 2015. "Impact of Community Interventions on the Social Representation of Depression in Rural Gujarat." *Psychiatric Quarterly* 86(3):419–433. doi: 10.1007/s11126-015-9342-x.

Moher, D., A. Liberati, J. Tetzlaff, and D. G. Altman. 2009. "Preferred Reporting Items for Systematic Reviews and Meta-Analyses: The PRISMA Statement." *PLoS Medicine* 6(7):e1000097. doi: 10.1371/journal.pmed.1000097.

Mosuro, S., D. Malcolm, and J. Guishard-Pine. 2014. "Mental Health Awareness and Coping in Foster Carers: The Impact of a Counselling Skills Intervention." *Educational & Child Psychology* 31(3):64–70.

Muscat, D. M., S. Smith, H. M. Dhillon, S. Morony, E. L. Davis, K. Luxford, H. L. Shepherd, A. Hayen, J. Comings, D. Nutbeam, and K. McCaffery. 2016. "Incorporating Health Literacy in Education for Socially Disadvantaged Adults: An Australian Feasibility Study." *International Journal for Equity in Health* 15:84. doi: 10.1186/s12939-016-0373-1.

Nagler, R. H., S. Ramanadhan, S. Minsky, and K. Viswanath. 2013. "Recruitment and Retention for Community-Based Ehealth Interventions with Populations of Low Socioeconomic Position: Strategies and Challenges." *Journal of Communication* 63(1):201–220. doi: 10.1111/jcom.12008.

Noble, J. M., M. G. Hedmann, and O. Williams. 2015. "Improving Dementia Health Literacy Using the FLOW Mnemonic: Pilot Findings from the Old SCHOOL Hip-Hop Program." *Health Education & Behavior* 42(1):73–83. doi: 10.1177/1090198114537063.

Nutbeam, D., B. McGill, and P. Premkumar. 2017. "Improving Health Literacy in Community Populations: A Review of Progress." *Health Promotion International*. doi: 10.1093/heapro/dax015.

Ohayon, J. L., E. Cousins, P. Brown, R. Morello-Frosch, and J. G. Brody. 2017. "Researcher and Institutional Review Board Perspectives on the Benefits and Challenges of Reporting Back Biomonitoring and Environmental Exposure Results." *Environmental Research* 153(February):140–149. doi: 10.1016/j.envres.2016.12.003.

Otilingam, P. G., M. Gatz, E. Tello, A. J. Escobar, A. Goldstein, M. Torres, and R. Varma. 2015. "Buenos Hábitos Alimenticios Para Una Buena Salud: Evaluation of a Nutrition Education Program to Improve Heart Health and Brain Health in Latinas." *Journal of Aging and Health* 27(1):177–192. doi: 10.1177/0898264314549660.

Ouzzani, M., H. Hammady, Z. Fedorowicz, and A. Elmagarmid. 2016. "Rayyan: A Web and Mobile App for Systematic Reviews." *Systematic Reviews* 5:210. doi: 10.1186/s13643-016-0384-4.

Oves, D. 2013. "Impact of Maternal Health Literacy Training on the Knowledge of Women Who Have Been Homeless." Power Point, Georgia State University. http://scholarworks.gsu.edu/iph_theses/304 (accessed June 1, 2017).

Pais, S. C., M. Rodrigues, and I. Menezes. 2014. "Community as Locus for Health Formal and Non-Formal Education: The Significance of Ecological and Collaborative Research for Promoting Health Literacy." *Frontiers in Public Health* 2. doi: 10.3389/fpubh.2014.00283.

Paul, M. P., P. Rigrod, S. Wingate, and M. E. Borsuk. 2015. "A Community-Driven Intervention in Tuftonboro, New Hampshire, Succeeds in Altering Water Testing Behavior." *Journal of Environmental Health* 78(5):30–39.

Pelto, D. J., G. R. Sadler, O. Njoku, M. C. Rodriguez, C. Villagra, V. L. Malcarne, N. E. Riley, A. I. Behar, and L. Jandorf. 2016. "Adaptation of a Cancer Clinical Trials Education Program for African American and Latina/o Community Members." *Health Education & Behavior* 43(4):381–388. doi: 10.1177/1090198115610555.

PHPartners. *About Partners: Partners in Information Access for the Public Health Workforce*. 2017. https://phpartners.org/about.html (accessed June 15, 2017).

Pinto-Foltz, M. D., M. C. Logsdon, and J. A. Myers. 2011. "Feasibility, Acceptability, and Initial Efficacy of a Knowledge-Contact Program to Reduce Mental Illness Stigma and Improve Mental Health Literacy in Adolescents." *Social Science & Medicine*, Part Special Issue: Analysing Global Health Assistance 72(12): 2011–2019. doi: 10.1016/j.socscimed.2011.04.006.

Pleasant, A. 2011. "Health Literacy: An Opportunity to Improve Individual, Community, and Global Health." *New Directions for Adult and Continuing Education* 2011(130):43–53. doi: 10.1002/ace.409.

Pomerantz, K. L., A. A. Muhammad, S. Downey, and T. Kind. 2010. "Connecting for Health Literacy: Health Information Partners." *Health Promotion Practice* 11(1):79–88. doi: 10.1177/1524839908318166.

Porter, K., Y. Chen, P. Estabrooks, L. Noel, A. Bailey, and J. Zoellner. 2016. "Using Teach-back to Understand Participant Behavioral Self-Monitoring Skills across Health Literacy Level and Behavioral Condition." *Journal of Nutrition Education and Behavior* 48(1):20–26. doi: 10.1016/j.jneb.2015.08.012.

Ramaswamy, M., R. Simmons, and P. J. Kelly. 2015. "The Development of a Brief Jail-Based Cervical Health Promotion Intervention." *Health Promotion Practice* 16(3):432–442. doi: 10.1177/1524839914541658.

Ramirez-Andreotta, M. D., J. G. Brody, N. Lothrop, M. Loh, P. I. Beamer, and P. Brown. 2016. "Improving Environmental Health Literacy and Justice through Environmental Exposure Results Communication." *International Journal of Environmental Research and Public Health* 13(7):690. doi: 10.3390/ijerph13070690.

Ramos, I. N., K. S. Ramos, A. Boerner, Q. He, and M. A. Tavera-Garcia. 2013. "Culturally-Tailored Education Programs to Address Health Literacy Deficits and Pervasive Health Disparities among Hispanics in Rural Shelbyville, Kentucky." *Journal of Community Medicine & Health Education* 3(7). doi: 10.4172/2161-0711.1000250.

Rexroth, D. F., and R. P. Friedland. 2010. "Lessons Learned Regarding Recruitment to the National African American Alzheimer Disease Health Literacy Program." *Alzheimer Disease and Associated Disorders* 24 Supplement(September):S54–S57.

Rodriguez, C. A. 2015. "A Fotonovela for Improving Dementia Literacy Among Latinos." Ph.D. dissertation, Los Angeles, CA: University of Southern California. http://search.proquest.com/docview/1767168864/abstract/F232DFE5703B488EPQ/1 (accessed June 1, 2017).

Romero, D. C., A. Sauris, F. Rodriguez, D. Delgado, A. Reddy, and J. M. Foody. 2016. "Vivir Con Un Corazón Saludable: A Community-Based Educational Program Aimed at Increasing Cardiovascular Health Knowledge in High-Risk Hispanic Women." *Journal of Racial and Ethnic Health Disparities* 3(1):99–107. doi: 10.1007/s40615-015-0119-6.

Rubin, D. L., V. S. Freimuth, S. D. Johnson, T. Kaley, and J. Parmer. 2014. "Training Meals on Wheels Volunteers as Health Literacy Coaches for Older Adults." *Health Promotion Practice* 15(3):448–454. doi: 10.1177/1524839913494786.

Rudd, R., L. Soricone, M. Santos, E. Zobel, and J. Smith. 2005. *Health Literacy Skills: Chronic Disease Management Study Circle + Guide.* Cambridge, MA: National Center for the Study of Adult Learning and Literacy (NCSALL). https://eric.ed.gov/?id=ED508597 (accessed June 1, 2017).

Sawilowsky, S. 2009. "New Effect Size Rules of Thumb." *Journal of Modern Applied Statistical Methods* 8(2). doi: 10.22237/jmasm/1257035100.

Schuster, A. L. R., K. D. Frick, B. Y. Huh, K. B. Kim, M. Kim, and H. R. Han. 2015. "Economic Evaluation of a Community Health Worker-Led Health Literacy Intervention to Promote Cancer Screening Among Korean American Women." *Journal of Health Care for the Poor and Underserved* 26(2):431–440. doi: 10.1353/hpu.2015.0050.

Selden, C. R., M. Zorn, S. Ratzan, and R. M. Parker. 2000. "Current Bibliographies in Medicine: Health Literacy." Bethesda, MD: National Library of Medicine. https://www.nlm.nih.gov/archive//20061214/pubs/cbm/hliteracy.html#10 (accessed June 1, 2017).

Shidhaye, R., V. Murhar, S. Gangale, L. Aldridge, R. Shastri, R. Parikh, R. Shrivastava, S. Damle, T. Raja, A. Nadkarni, and V. Patel. 2017. "The Effect of VISHRAM, a Grass-Roots Community-Based Mental Health Programme, on the Treatment Gap for Depression in Rural Communities in India: A Population-Based Study." *The Lancet Psychiatry* 4(2):128–135. doi: 10.1016/S2215-0366(16)30424-2.

Shreffler-Grant, J., E. G. Nichols, and C. Weinert. 2017. "Bee SAFE, a Skill-Building Intervention to Enhance CAM Health Literacy: Lessons Learned." *Health Promotion Practice* April, 1524839917700612. doi: 10.1177/1524839917700612.

Son, J., W. M. Miller, K. Tossone, F. Butcher, and K. Kuo. 2017. "The Effect of Interprofessional Student-Led Reproductive Health Education on Youths in Juvenile Detention." *Journal of Pediatric and Adolescent Gynecology* 30(3):370–375. doi: 10.1016/j.jpag.2016.11.002.

Soto Mas, F., C. Cordova, A. Murrietta, H. Jacobson, F. Ronquillo, and D. Helitzer. 2015. "A Multisite Community-Based Health Literacy Intervention for Spanish Speakers." *Journal of Community Health* 40(3):431–438. doi: 10.1007/s10900-014-9953-4.

Soto Mas, F., M. Ji, B. O. Fuentes, and J. Tinajero. 2015. "The Health Literacy and ESL Study: A Community-Based Intervention for Spanish-Speaking Adults." *Journal of Health Communication* 20(4):369–376. doi: 10.1080/10810730.2014.965368.

Spencer, L. M., M. W. Schooley, L. A. Anderson, C. S. Kochtitzky, A. S. DeGroff, H. M. Devlin, and S. L. Mercer. 2013. "Seeking Best Practices: A Conceptual Framework for Planning and Improving Evidence-Based Practices." *Preventing Chronic Disease* 10 (December): E207. doi: 10.5888/pcd10.130186.

Stockwell, M., M. Catallozzi, D. Meyer, C. Rodriguez, E. Martinez, and E. Larson. 2010. "Improving Care of Upper Respiratory Infections Among Latino Early Head Start Parents." *Journal of Immigrant & Minority Health* 12(6):925–931. doi: 10.1007/s10903-010-9326-8.

Svensson, B., L. Hansson, and S. Stjernswärd. 2015. "Experiences of a Mental Health First Aid Training Program in Sweden: A Descriptive Qualitative Study." *Community Mental Health Journal* 51(4):497–503. doi: 10.1007/s10597-015-9840-1.

Taylor, K. A., M. A. Lindeman, K. Stothers, K. Piper, and P. Kuipers. 2012. "Intercultural Communications in Remote Aboriginal Australian Communities: What Works in Dementia Education and Management?" *Health Sociology Review; Abingdon* 21(2):208–219.

Tuerk, P. W., B. Hall, N. Nagae, J. L. McCauley, M. Yoder, S. A. M. Rauch, R. Acierno, and J. Dussich. 2013. "Forty Days After the Great East Japan Earthquake: Field Research Investigating Community Engagement and Traumatic Stress Screening in a Post-Disaster Community Mental Health Training." *The International Journal of Psychiatry in Medicine* 45(2):159–174. doi: 10.2190/PM.45.2.e.

Unger, J. B., L. J. Cabassa, G. B. Molina, S. Contreras, and M. Baron. 2013. "Evaluation of a Fotonovela to Increase Depression Knowledge and Reduce Stigma among Hispanic Adults." *Journal of Immigrant and Minority Health* 15(2):398–406. doi: 10.1007/s10903-012-9623-5.

Vanderbilt, A. A., M. S. Wright, A. E. Brewer, L. K. Murithi, and P. Coney. 2016. "Increasing Knowledge and Health Literacy about Preterm Births in Underserved Communities: An Approach to Decrease Health Disparities, a Pilot Study." *Global Journal of Health Science* 8(1):83–89. doi: 10.5539/gjhs.v8n1p83.

Vollmer Dahlke, D., K. Fair, Y.A. Hong, D. Kellstedt, and M.G. Ory. 2017. "Adolescent and Young Adult Cancer Survivorship Educational Programming: A Qualitative Evaluation." *JMIR Cancer* 3(1):e3. doi: 10.2196/cancer.5821.

Weiss, B. D., M. Z. Mays, W. Martz, K. Merriam Castro, D. A. DeWalt, M. P. Pignone, J. Mockbee, and F. A. Hale. 2005. "Quick Assessment of Literacy in Primary Care: The Newest Vital Sign." *The Annals of Family Medicine* 3(6):514–522. doi: 10.1370/afm.405.

White, A., J. South, A. M. Bagnall, M. Forshaw, C. Spoor, P. Marchant, and K. Witty. 2012. "The Self-Care for People Initiative: The Outcome Evaluation." *Primary Health Care Research & Development* 13(4):382–394. doi: 10.1017/S146342361200014X.

Williams, M. V., D. W. Baker, R. M. Parker, and J. R. Nurss. 1998. "Relationship of Functional Health Literacy to Patients' Knowledge of Their Chronic Disease: A Study of Patients with Hypertension and Diabetes." *Archives of Internal Medicine* 158(2):166–172. doi: 10.1001/archinte.158.2.166.

Wong, D. F. K., Y. Lau, S. Kwok, P. Wong, and C. Tori. 2017. "Evaluating the Effectiveness of Mental Health First Aid Program for Chinese People in Hong Kong." *Research on Social Work Practice* 27(1):59–67. doi: 10.1177/1049731515585149.

Wood, A.L. and O.F. Wahl. 2006. "Evaluating the Effectiveness of a Consumer-Provided Mental Health Recovery Education Presentation." *Psychiatric Rehabilitation* 30(1):46–53. doi: 10.2975/30.2006.46.53.

Xie, B. 2011. "Improving Older Adults' E-Health Literacy Through Computer Training Using NIH Online Resources." *Library & Information Science Research* 34(1):63–71. doi: 10.1016/j.lisr.2011.07.006.

Zhuang, R., Y. Xiang, T. Han, G. A. Yang, and Y. Zhang. 2016. "Cell Phone-Based Health Education Messaging Improves Health Literacy." *African Health Sciences* 16(1):311–318. doi: 10.4314/ahs.v16i1.41.